EXERCISE
THE BEST HEALTH
INSURANCE

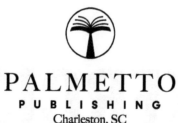

PALMETTO
P U B L I S H I N G
Charleston, SC
www.PalmettoPublishing.com

Hardcover ISBN: 979-8-8229-5299-7
Paperback ISBN: 979-8-8229-4240-0
eBook ISBN: 979-8-8229-4241-7

EXERCISE
THE BEST HEALTH
INSURANCE

TRANFORMING HEALTH
AND REDUCING COSTS
THROUGH ACTIVE LIVING

WISLER SAINT-VIL, MD, MBA

AUTHOR AFFILIATIONS

Sports medicine medical director at Memorial Health System, Marietta, Ohio

Clinical faculty in family medicine and emergency medicine at Memorial Health System, Marietta, Ohio

Former sports medicine fellow physician for the Cleveland Browns, National Football League

Founder of ExerciseNow, an EMR-integrated sports medicine platform

Founder of the Haitian Vision Foundation, a nonprofit organization dedicated to health care and education initiatives

Member of the American Medical Society for Sports Medicine, contributing to the advancement of sports medicine through research and practice

Member of the American College of Sports Medicine, committed to improving health through sports and physical activity

Member of the American Academy of Family Physicians, promoting high-quality, comprehensive health care

Member of the American Medical Association, advocating for the interests and professionalism of medical doctors and the improvement of public health

DEDICATION

This book is dedicated to the following:

To my loving parents, who believed in me from the beginning and never wavered in supporting my dreams. This book is a tribute to you for nurturing my aspirations.

To my spouse, Asiane Saint-Vil, you are my rock and muse. Your unwavering love and faith in me have been the guiding light throughout this writing journey. This book is a testament to our bond.

To the readers who embark on this journey with me, who get lost in the pages, finding solace, joy, or a new perspective, this book is dedicated to you for your unwavering support and for embracing the worlds I have created.

To the teachers and mentors who have shaped me as a writer and encouraged me to pursue my passion, your guidance and wisdom have made all the difference. This book honors your invaluable contributions.

To my dear colleague Dr. Timothy Graham, your unwavering encouragement has been a constant source of inspiration. Thank you for always being there and pushing me to reach new heights.

Last, I dedicate this to my children, Astin and Ashmene, whose presence in my life has fueled my determination to pursue my dreams relentlessly. May this book serve as a beacon, inspiring you to explore the boundless possibilities of your mind.

CONTENTS

Author Bio 1

Preface 5

Module I: Exercise and Health 9

Lack of Exercise Is the Single Most Important

Cause of Health Disorders 12

Exercise and Mortality 16

Exercise and Disability 21

Quality of life (QoL) and Exercise 26

End-of-Module-I Activities 32

End-of-Module Quiz 37

Answers 39

Module II: Exercise Types and Their Benefits 41

Aerobic and Cardio 42

Strength and Resistance Training 48

HIIT 52

Stretching Exercises 57

Sports Training 62

Yoga and Pilates 64

Exercises for Rehabilitation and Recovery 67

End-of-Module-II Activities 70

End-of-Module Quiz 75

Answers 77

Module III: Tips for Getting Started with Exercise 79

Assess Your Fitness Level 81

Create Your Fitness Program 85

Invest in Equipment and a New Lifestyle 89

Get Started 89

Keep Monitoring 91

The Triangle of Success 92

Keep Learning and Improving Your Technique 94

End-of-Module-III Activities 96

End-of-Module Quiz 101

Answers 103

Module IV: How Exercise Helps Curb Appetite 105

End-of-Module-IV Activities 116

End-of-Module Quiz 121

Answers 123

Module V: Benefits of Regular Physical Activity 125

Weight Control 126

Reduces Risk of Chronic Health Conditions and Diseases 131

Improves Mood 136

Boosts Energy Levels 142

Promotes Better Sleep 144

Brings Back the Spark to Your Sex Life 147

It's Fun and Helps One Socialize 153

Exercise Is the Best Antiaging Medicine 155

Exercise Helps Prevent Cognitive Decline 158

Good for Bone Health 161

Helps Reverse or Treat Disease Conditions 164

Increases Self-Esteem and Helps One Look Good 169

The Bottom Line on Exercise 172

End-of-Module-V Activities 176

End-of-Module Quiz 181

Answers 183

Module VI: Health Insurance 185

Types of Health Insurance 188

Public Health Care Coverage 189

Private Health Coverage 191

Types of Medical Insurance 194

End-of-Module-VI Activities 198

End-of-Module Quiz 202

Answers 204

Module VII: Health Insurance Companies Are Tracking Your Data 205

End-of-Module-VII Activities 212

End-of-Module Quiz 217

Answers 219

Module VIII: Life and Health 221

Lower Your Insurance and Medical Expenses with

Diet and Exercise 225

End-of-Module-VIII Activities 233

End-of-Module Quiz 238

Answers: 240

References 241

Acknowledgments 248

AUTHOR BIO

Dr. Wisler Saint-Vil is a fellowship-trained sports medicine physician, a renowned researcher, and an innovative leader in health care. He has dedicated his career to treating sports injuries across a diverse range of athletes and individuals of all ages, including professional athletes and those with various musculoskeletal conditions.

Dr. Saint-Vil significantly advanced in this field during his distinguished Sports Medicine Fellowship at Case Western Reserve University under the aegis of University Hospitals Cleveland Medical Center. He served as a fellow physician for esteemed teams and institutions, including the Cleveland Browns, Kent State University, Lake Erie College, Case Western Reserve University, and various Cleveland area high schools. This diverse experience not only honed his medical skills but also deepened his understanding of the unique needs and challenges faced by athletes across different levels of sports.

As medical director for the Marietta Memorial Hospital Sports Medicine department, Dr. Saint-Vil also leads as a team physician for Marietta College and more than ten high schools in the Mid-Ohio Valley and West Virginia. His expertise extends beyond his sports medicine background and is driven by a personal history as a former athlete, giving him unique insights into the challenges and recovery processes of sports-related injuries.

Dr. Saint-Vil's commitment to improving health care extends to his academic pursuits. He specializes in minimally invasive regenerative medicine, focusing on innovative treatments like platelet rich plasma and percutaneous needle tenotomy. His academic interests include the use of platelet rich plasma in regenerating tendons, ligaments, cartilage, and soft tissues, and he is a published author in notable journals and magazines.

Recognizing the need for broader systemic improvements in patient care and health care management, Dr. Saint-Vil pursued an Executive MBA at the Haslam College of Business, University of Tennessee. This endeavor was fueled by his passion for revolutionizing the health care system; he aims to integrate his medical expertise with advanced business strategies to enhance patient care on a larger scale.

Dr. Saint-Vil is fluent in English, Spanish, French, and Haitian Creole, and his multilingual abilities reflect his experience working in multicultural environments and his commitment to accessible, inclusive patient care. His holistic approach to medicine, combined with his educational background and leadership skills, positions him at the forefront of health care innovation and patient advocacy.

PREFACE

This book primarily explains why everyone must be exercising in the first place and why it is essential, not an option. It also discusses the health benefits of various exercise forms and provides a detailed road map for getting started. There is much focus on how it may help improve health and prevent many health disorders, with some discussion about the underlying mechanism—thus explaining why exercise is the best health insurance.

This book does not provide any exercise plan as one size does not fit all and people need to have an individualized plan. In addition, the plan depends on age, health status, and other factors.

Of course, this book is about health insurance too. There is a discussion about various insurance options and how to exercise to stay healthy and reduce your health insurance premiums. In addition, this book tries to show people multiple technologies that insurance companies use to track their health, thus deciding how much a person must pay for insurance.

Thinking about insurance is beneficial and saving on insurance is necessary to avoid spending time working for insurance premiums. Instead, spend that time doing something you enjoy. However, the primary focus of any exercise must be improving health as the rest will all follow automatically, including good health, perfect body shape, increased energy level, joy, and saving on insurance premiums.

Many books and websites discuss diet and how to improve health through diet. A lot of materials explain how to exercise and get beach-ready. Most of those materials are provided by health experts and self-made gurus. However, these materials, books, websites, and podcasts place less focus on explaining how exercise can actually boost your health and prevent diseases. This book takes a scientific approach to the subject. Though it is not a comprehensive guide or a medical textbook, it tries to be as accurate as possible.

If you exercise, you won't need to switch to restrictive diets, as that may not be a healthy option. Exercise can alter your mental health and mood and influence your choices. It will result in better sleep, for sure.

The three most important things people must do to stay healthy and enjoy life are to move a lot or exercise, eat a balanced diet, and sleep sufficiently. However, if you do not exercise, implementing dietary measures or improving sleep is challenging.

To understand the importance of exercise, we need to consider human evolution. Humans evolved to engage in physical labor, earn their sustenance through hard work, and then enjoy restful nights. However, advancements in technology and subsequent changes in lifestyle have disrupted this natural balance. People no longer need to engage in physical labor to secure their meals; there is an abundance of food, and sleep patterns have been altered. Additionally, sunlight no longer dictates our daily routines.

Nonetheless, incorporating exercise into our lives can gradually and naturally restore this equilibrium, leading to overall improvements in various aspects of our well-being.

For example, the restrictive diets that many are recommending are not the right way to health. If you give up that many foods, it causes not only stress but also malnutrition in the long term. In addition, a body that is not eating properly and not moving enough cannot be expected to sleep well or have a pain-free life.

If we closely examine the developments of the past century, we observe a sudden shift toward a more sedentary lifestyle, marked by decreased physical activity and mobility. The human body is designed to conserve resources by reducing support to underutilized systems and organs, driven by negative feedback mechanisms. Consequently, this leads to various adverse effects, including the weakening of the heart, muscle atrophy, joint deterioration, and even a decline in the function of organs such as the liver.

So, if you want to enjoy life to the fullest, you must be moving and exercising. The rest will follow. You will be in better shape and have a normal body weight, fine-tuned metabolism, disease-free body, and stress- and depression-free brain. You will eliminate your food addiction, start eating healthy foods, and improve your sleep. This book will teach you how exercise can transform your life and why it is the best health insurance.

MODULE I

EXERCISE AND HEALTH

B eginning a regular exercise routine is arguably the most crucial step you can take toward enhancing your health, remaining free from illness, and embracing happiness. Engaging in physical activity not only promises a life with reduced pain but also offers significant financial benefits, particularly in terms of reducing health care costs. It's essential to understand that exercise is more than just a physical activity—it's a proactive investment in your well-being. In essence, "exercise is the best health insurance."

This book is designed to be your guide and companion on this journey. It provides you with the necessary tools and knowledge to initiate your exercise regimen, maintain consistency, and enjoy the rewards of a vigorous, healthful lifestyle. By following the insights and strategies within these pages, you can look forward to not only substantial savings on health insurance expenses but also a life brimming with activity and vitality.

Health experts now call a sedentary lifestyle the most important cause of health disorders. They call it "a new kind of smoking," as the harms of a sedentary lifestyle are no less than those of smoking. There is nothing that can replace the benefits of exercise: no dietary measures, pills, or supplements.

One must look back in time to understand why exercise is vital for humans. Look back hundreds or even thousands of years. For this, one needs to understand how humans have evolved.

We humans have reached this stage of evolution by hunting and gathering, engaging in physical activity most of the day, all the year around. Yes, we did use our brains all the time, but we also kept moving.

If you have any doubts about the physical abilities of humans, then stop and think. Humans are among the fastest-running bipeds. Here, keep in mind that the ostrich is a bird. So among mammals, perhaps the kangaroo is the only mammal that can run faster than us on two legs.

However, humans can outrun most mammals due to their high endurance. In terms of endurance, humans are closer to wolves. The cheetah gets tired in just a few minutes, and even the lion cannot run for long. On the other hand, humans can readily run for a few miles, and trained bodies can run tens of miles.

So the human body evolved to work physically for long hours and then, after sunset, have a sound sleep.

But everything suddenly started to change abruptly at the dawn of the twentieth century, when the industrial age was in full swing. It was the time when a considerable number of humans started to engage in work that did not require much physical movement. Industry needed investors, managers, clerks, salespeople, and more.

Things became worse with the advent of the information age, and now most people are stuck at their desks in front of a screen. As a result, even their entertainment habits have changed.

Such changes have led to a sedentary lifestyle. For example, instead of hunting or playing outdoor games, people would rather watch television.

Lack of Exercise Is the Single Most Important Cause of Health Disorders

One might think, What is wrong with sitting or lying down for a long time? After all, it provides pleasure and it is something humans have been dreaming of for a long time. Humans have dreamed of a comfortable lifestyle, security, and abundant food. It appears that they have achieved all of this to a significant extent.

So what could possibly be wrong with sitting and enjoying oneself? Humans, after all, do not need the kind of endurance they needed a few centuries back.

Well, there are some vital reasons to keep moving and to start exercising. Unlike the common misbelief, lack of exercise may not significantly reduce your lifespan. After all, medicine has progressed a lot. However, a lack of exercise increases one's risk for various diseases. In addition, it results in higher expenditure on insurance and thus a need to work for longer hours. This will ultimately beat the whole purpose of staying in the comfort zone for too long and not moving.

Getting treated for various disorders is not a pleasant task, nor is working long hours to pay for health insurance. On the other hand, one can choose a physical activity of their liking, significantly reduce the risk of diseases, and significantly reduce health insurance payments.

Even health experts, researchers, and doctors have found it difficult to understand the significance of exercise for good health. For decades, they have been wondering, finding it almost impossible to explain the increase in specific health disorders.

Science continues to struggle to understand why so many people develop heart disease at an early age. Likewise, why are so many people developing diabetes?

Perhaps the significant rise of diseases like Alzheimer's and mental health disorders has come as an even greater surprise. No one imagined that rare conditions like dementia would become the leading cause of disability and death.

However, researchers have noticed that these days, people are more likely to die of noncommunicable (noninfectious) diseases like heart attack, stroke, diabetes (and its complications), dementia, and more.[1] Thus, they started asking many questions and they found the reply. All their findings showed that lack of exercise is the most significant contributor to the rise of these disorders.

Health experts and researchers analyzed various factors. For example, it is pretty simple to conclude that human genetics have not changed much in the last century. However, our environment, dietary habits, and lifestyle have considerably changed.[2]

Humans are now exposed to more toxins, but this is insufficient to explain the health problems people face. Moreover, people living in relatively good or healthy environments also develop various chronic health disorders at a young age. So toxins could be a contributing factor but are not a major factor.

Diet, on the other hand, has improved, and malnutrition is rare in developed nations like the US or EU Zone. These days, people in developed economies are more likely to develop diseases due to excessive calorie intake rather than malnutrition. So, yes, diet contributes to the increase in illnesses. However, dietary changes are not sufficient to escape many health problems.

Finally, experts have turned their attention to the level of physical activity, which has significantly declined. Yes, people might be busy at work, but that is not considered physical activity. It is rather a source of mental stress.

Studies show that people are just not moving enough, which is perhaps the leading cause of all health disorders. This weakens the heart, respiratory system, immunity, and musculoskeletal system and negatively affects almost every body function. It even results in greater mental stress.

Moreover, it is pretty easy to understand that changing one's environment is challenging and not possible in many cases. Adapting to new environments can make maintaining an exercise routine difficult, with challenges such as limited access to safe exercise spaces, varying weather conditions, and busy lifestyles. These factors necessitate the need for flexible and accessible fitness solutions that cater to individual circumstances. Dieting is not an option, as reducing food intake would increase the risk of malnutrition.

So what is the way out?

Exercise is the best way to stay healthy, burn calories, fine-tune every body organ, and stay fit and healthy. And ultimately, it helps cut down insurance costs, as we've already discussed. It will even translate into spending fewer hours working and more time enjoying your life.

Exercise and Mortality

Perhaps the most important motivator for exercise is that it prolongs life. When doctors tell people that by exercising, they can expect to live a few years longer or even extend their life by a few decades, that is highly motivating.

By talking about long life and prolonged existence, doctors are exploiting the power of the most basic human instinct—the instinct of survival.

But does exercise really prolong life? Can it realistically add a few years to life? Well, yes, most studies suggest that is the case. In addition, exercise can considerably lower the mortality rate.

To understand to what degree physical activity can extend your life, you need to look at some of the statistics.

According to the CDC (Center for Disease Control), the leading causes of mortality in the US in 2021 were:[1]

1. Heart disease
2. Cancer
3. COVID-19
4. Accidents (unintentional injuries)
5. Stroke (cerebrovascular diseases)

6. Chronic lower respiratory diseases

7. Alzheimer's disease

8. Diabetes

9. Influenza and pneumonia

10. Nephritis, nephrotic syndrome, and nephrosis

As one can see in the list above, most of these are noninfectious diseases. Therefore, exercise has a significant benefit in reducing mortality related to noninfectious diseases. However, remember that regular exercise can also significantly reduce the risk of infection-related death.

Just consider conditions like heart disease, stroke, and chronic lower respiratory conditions. These are diseases that are highly preventable through exercise. In many cases, it may reduce your risk of developing these ailments by almost half.

Of course, one might ask, What if someone has a family history of heart disease? In such cases, exercise still helps significantly. Instead of having a first heart attack at the age of 50 or 60, one may have a minor heart problem at the age of 70 or 80. That is a significant difference.

Exercise can benefit people in the most unexpected ways. For example, physically trained people are less likely to abuse substances, smoke, and alcohol and thus are less likely to have motor vehicle accidents.

Similarly, a physically trained individual is less likely to fall and suffer severe and life-threatening injuries.

There is sufficient data to show that physically active people are less likely to develop cancer; indeed, one can readily add a few years to their life through exercise.

Diabetes has a direct relation to faulty food choices and a sedentary lifestyle. Therefore, dietary corrections and extensive physical activity can help prevent diabetes in most instances. Not only that, but it can even help reverse diabetes in some cases.[3]

One might think, OK, that is fine, but can exercise reduce mortality risk due to COVID-19 and influenza? The answer here is yes. Exercises boost cardiorespiratory fitness, and survival depends on cardiorespiratory fitness when one catches a respiratory infection. Moreover, metabolic health also plays a significant role in survivability, and exercise is the best way to boost metabolic health.

When it comes to kidney diseases, these disorders are almost always secondary to diabetes and cardiovascular ailments. Thus, one can see that exercise can even ensure renal health. Moreover, exercise improves diuresis, detoxification, and kidney health in many other ways.[4]

Here, it is also vital to understand the interrelationship between various ailments. A step taken to prevent one kind of noninfectious disease helps significantly reduce the risk of other ailments and thus prolong life.

One does not need to do different kinds of exercise to prevent various diseases and prolong life. However, it is essential to get started and keep going. Exercise boosts cardiorespiratory health, immunity, and metabolic health and prevents most of these disorders.

Of course, exercise is not a magic pill, and people are not immortal. So what we are suggesting is that exercise can delay life-threatening conditions and even aging. In most cases, it can delay these unpleasant events by years and even decades.

Many are skeptical of such claims. Some still disbelieve the health benefits of exercise. They might say that they know someone who exercised and yet had some severe health issues. However, remember, as we already stated, exercise will either delay or prevent disease but will not make anyone immortal.

Another vital factor to know is something called the "legacy effect." It refers to the fact that the earlier you start exercising, the greater the benefit.

That said, many people neglect their health for years. As a result, they accumulate tens of pounds of fat. Then, suddenly, they join a boot camp, start exercising, and become lean.

These individuals may look good, healthy, and lean, but they need time to eliminate the negative consequences of years of neglect. In other words, they need *time to overcome the legacy effect.*[5]

This does not mean that starting exercise late in life or after developing ailments will not help. On the contrary, exercise helps in every case. However, it helps less when you start exercising too late.

Don't expect that years of neglect to not have any long-lasting ill effects. Exercise can help overcome those issues, but it takes more time. The ill effects of twenty years of a sedentary lifestyle, substance abuse, and being overweight cannot be erased in a year, but one can neutralize them in a few years.

Here, it is also vital to understand that if someone looks good and has a chiseled body, it does not mean that person is metabolically healthy. The primary goal of exercise must be to become fit from the inside.

It is never too late to start, so if you want to prolong your life and prevent untimely severe health issues, today is the best day to get started. It does not matter what kind of physical activity you engage in; all sorts of exercises are going to help. Still, a well-planned exercise regime will have more significant benefits.

Exercise and Disability

It is not sufficient to have a long life. As already mentioned, medical care and drug therapy alone can contribute to a long life. In fact, improved medical care has contributed to greater life expectancy, more so than any other factor.

So, yes, exercise is not just about prolonging life. It is even more about reducing disability. As we've seen, many, many health conditions won't kill you but will cause significant disability.

Think of a condition like osteoarthritis. It rarely kills. But just imagine living with painful joints for thirty years. That is not to frighten you, as such pain is a fact of life for many. Unfortunately, more and more people are being affected by severe osteoarthritis at a relatively young age. Exercise is the single most effective way to delay these health issues.

Before we dive deeper into the subject, let's just revisit the list of leading causes of death in the US. Here is an important question everyone must be asking themselves: Do those diseases always kill instantly, or do they cause years of disability?

If you are unsure, think of a person with an aching heart or someone who survived a stroke but cannot walk and speak normally. Or think of a person living with dementia. Most people with Alzheimer's die a slow death, spending years or even a decade with a disability, high medical bills, insurance payments—the list goes on.[6]

Similarly, think of diabetes. It never kills anyone instantly. Most people diagnosed with type 2 diabetes can expect to live several decades. However, they will need continuous treatment and be exposed to high insurance payments.

Not only that, but diabetes is also the leading cause of foot amputation, chronic kidney disease, retinopathy, neuropathy, and other painful conditions. This means that though medications extend life, they do not nullify suffering or disability.[7]

Living with a disability, working, and paying insurance bills can be pretty painful. In addition, working to pay insurance bills is not an activity anyone wants to engage in.

Again, exercise can help prevent these issues. For example, if a person has a heart issue later in life, they are less likely to live with a disability for a long time. Additionally, physically active individuals are more likely to recover fully after severe issues like an accident.

The importance of exercise in preventing disability is frequently overlooked in discussions. People don't just aim to prolong their lives; they also want to enjoy a pain-free existence and avoid the financial burden of constant medical bills. Consequently, we should emphasize that disability prevention is a significant and essential benefit of incorporating regular exercise into one's life.

Studies show that exercise can not only prevent debilitating conditions but can also reverse them. Exercise can be the best treatment for many health conditions. Once one is diagnosed with diabetes, high blood pressure, high cholesterol, or even arthritis, the first thing they should think of is to start exercising.

Regretfully, many people find it easier to start taking pills. We are not suggesting that one should not take pills. What we are saying is that pills are not a replacement for exercise. Medical drugs or health supplements may help, but they rarely reverse a disability as effectively as physical activity.

Think of physiotherapy. Everyone knows its value in rehabilitation, yet it remains a neglected medical field. People with chronic pain are happily taking opioids, which further aggravates their health problem, instead of considering physiotherapy.

Physiotherapy is a kind of exercise therapy prescribed in a more controlled manner. It involves prescribing more specific physical movements for faster recovery from specific health conditions. Again, it helps, though it requires much effort.

Before we move on to the next topic, it is vital to touch on another important factor, which is the role of exercise in reducing **mental health disabilities**.[8]

Mental health disorders like anxiety and depression are among the leading causes of disability. Exercise is not just about boosting physical health; it can also significantly improve mental health. Further, exercise is not just about building endurance, lean mass, and so on. It is also about reducing stress and improving cognitive function.

Those who exercise regularly are less likely to develop mental health disorders. Not only that, but they are also less likely to suffer from age-related cognitive decline.

If you exercise, you will have less time to worry about unessential things. Not only that, but it will also alter your brain health. So for many, starting to exercise can be a life-changing experience.

Exercise also entails increased release of endorphins, and from this, one experiences greater pleasure from life and various activities. Those with adequate endorphins are less likely to seek happiness by abusing substances.

Further, remember that exercise is not just about hitting the gym or lifting heavy weights. An enjoyable evening walk counts as exercise, just like swimming or playing your favorite sports.

In fact, it is a pretty simple fact that the fewer steps we take in a day, the faster we age and the more likely we are to develop some disability. This is the reason why most wearable technologies pay so much attention to the number of steps taken in a day; it could be the single most important measurement of good health.

A greater number of daily steps ultimately translates into better health, longer life, reduced disability, lower medical bills, and lower health insurance payments. Thus, exercise is for disability prevention, staying active, and enjoying life.

Did we say "enjoying life"? Yes, without health, you cannot do that. And that is the next topic of discussion. Doctors or health experts may talk about disease prevention, prolonging life, and reducing disability, but they rarely speak about the fun side of life.

What is the sense of living a life that lacks fun? And yes, exercise can add that fun to your life. In medical language, we say it can increase quality of life (QoL).

Quality of life (QoL) and Exercise

The reason I exercise is for the quality of life I enjoy.
—Kenneth H. Cooper

A person might well live for a long time and not suffer from any disability—this is, in fact, the case for a significant number of people. However, this does not necessarily mean the individuals in question are feeling well and enjoying life to the fullest.

It is unwise to view exercise only as something that prolongs your health and prevents diseases. Indeed, the absence of disease does not even mean that a person is well.

In recent years, the concept of wellness has emerged, and experts have come to understand that health and wellness are quite different. Although most people may be healthy at any given moment, this does not mean they are feeling well.

Many people keep complaining about a lack of mood and energy, feeling unwell, and not feeling like engaging in any activity. Yet in physical and lab examinations, doctors cannot find any health issues. Nor do these people have a mental health disorder.

It appears that exercise and greater engagement in physical activities might be one of the most effective ways of feeling well. Feeling well is directly related to QoL.[9]

QoL is an even broader term than wellness. It is the ultimate goal of life to have a higher QoL. Even if you are disease-free, lack any disability, and feel well, you are not necessarily enjoying your life.

Exercise provides you with the much-needed vigor required to enjoy your life to the fullest. Of course, these changes may not occur in a day. But regular physical activity ensures an excellent quality of life. It means a greater degree of socializing, adequate sexual desire and function, and increased engagement in various activities. Good health ensures that one can achieve everything needed for QoL, like securing wealth, a job, physical and mental health, wellness, education, the ability to participate in recreational activities, social belonging, security, freedom, and the ability to spend one's leisure time as one wishes.

Although QoL is quite a broad concept, it is worthwhile to explore and understand it to achieve happiness in life.

For example, regular exercise enables you to stay healthy and have a better intimate relationship with your partner. As a result, you may have a better sex life, travel together more often, engage in various activities together, and thus have a higher level of life satisfaction.

Similarly, these days, most people have their first child when they are older than thirty. This means that by the time their child is a teenager, they are already close to fifty years of age. Regular exercise can help adults stay active and engage more with their children, thus achieving a higher QoL.

Consider another example: You decide to go to the mountains or some national park. The best places or spots there are inaccessible by car or bike, and the only way to reach them is on foot. Hence, your ability to enjoy your holiday depends on your physical training and how much you exercise. The more you walk and travel, the happier you are and the higher your QoL.

It is not rare to see people visiting mountains, national parks, and other places of natural beauty and then struggling to move and enjoy themselves. Even worse, many people develop some kind of sickness whenever they go to new places or on holidays. These are seemingly healthy people with no disease or disability, yet they have low QoL as they are just unfit to enjoy the pleasures of life provided to us by Mother Nature.

There is a reason why we are focusing so much on QoL here: it is among the less-often-discussed concepts in health care. Your doctor is not going to discuss it with you. They will mostly focus on the health benefits of exercise and how it may help prevent or manage ailments.

Further, as we've discussed, most people visiting doctors are more interested in getting treated for their presenting condition through medical drugs. Regretfully, doctors lack time to explain the broader benefits of exercise, benefits beyond good health.

Therefore, exercise should not be considered merely a tool that prolongs life or prevents disability. Indeed, medications can prolong life, and doctors can also treat disabilities. However, your QoL only depends on you and your physical and mental well-being.

Exercise is one of the most effective ways of improving your QoL. Moreover, improved QoL is perhaps one of the most significant benefits of engaging in regular exercise.

By developing a better understanding of how exercise and increased physical activity can transform every aspect of life, we can stop looking at exercise as physical exertion causing pain and fatigue. Although getting started with exercise may be challenging, as you progress, you will realize that all the pain and sweat it causes are worth it.

So let exercise be your new and only addiction. It is the only known healthy addiction, one that opens the road to good health, wellness, and happiness.

Exercise not only contributes to cost savings on health insurance, but it is, in itself, a form of health insurance. Unlike traditional medical insurance, this type of insurance demands a relatively modest investment in the form of effort and sweat. In return, you can anticipate substantial dividends for your health and well-being.

Since you now know the real benefits of exercising, you must be wondering where to start. What kind of exercise is best for you?

Though any exercise is better than no exercise, there are many distinct types of physical activity, all with their own health benefits. In addition, some forms of exercise may be better choices for you. So, let's explore various exercise types and their benefits together.

END-OF-MODULE-I ACTIVITIES

Personal Reflection: Take a moment to reflect on your current exercise habits. Are you a beginner, intermediate, or advanced in terms of fitness? What are your main fitness goals?

_____

_____

_____

_____

_____

_____

_____

_____

_____

_____

_____

_____

_____

Activity Planner: Based on your fitness level and goals, create a weekly exercise plan. Include a variety of exercises, such as cardio, strength training, and flexibility exercises. Remember to consider your schedule and be realistic about the time you can dedicate.

_____

_____

_____

_____

_____

_____

_____

_____

_____

_____

_____

_____

Implementation: Follow your exercise plan for a week. Take note of how you feel before and after each session. Are there any changes in your mood, energy levels, or sleep patterns?

_____

_____

_____

_____

_____

_____

_____

_____

_____

_____

_____

_____

_____

_____

Journaling: Keep a daily journal of your activities. Record the type of exercise, duration, and your feelings about each session. Also, note any barriers you faced in sticking to your plan and how you overcame them.

_____

_____

_____

_____

_____

_____

_____

_____

_____

_____

_____

_____

_____

Reflection and Adjustment: At the end of the week, review your journal. Reflect on what worked well and what didn't. Adjust your plan for the next week based on this reflection.

_____

_____

_____

_____

_____

_____

_____

_____

_____

_____

_____

_____

_____

_____

_____

_____

END-OF-MODULE QUIZ

1. **Question:** What is the primary benefit of regular physical activity?

   A) It only helps in weight loss.

   B) It improves mood and energy levels.

   C) It increases the risk of chronic diseases.

   D) It is only for professional athletes.

2. **Question:** How does exercise impact the risk of noncommunicable diseases?

   A) Increases the risk

   B) No impact

   C) Reduces the risk

   D) Only affects communicable diseases

3. **Question:** What role does exercise play in quality of life (QoL)?

   A) No role

   B) Decreases QoL

   C) Increases QoL

   D) Only affects physical appearance

4. **Question:** True or False: Exercise can only improve physical health, not mental health.

A) True

B) False

5. **Question:** What is the "legacy effect" in the context of exercise?

A) The impact of exercise on future generations

B) The historical importance of exercise

C) The benefits of exercise accumulating over time

D) The influence of past exercises on current health

ANSWERS

1. B) It improves mood and energy levels.

2. C) Reduces the risk

3. C) Increases QoL

4. B) False

5. C) The benefits of exercise accumulating over time

MODULE II

EXERCISE TYPES AND THEIR BENEFITS

There are a few different exercise types, and they have different health benefits. The choice of exercise type depends on many factors, such as health conditions and objectives. For example, some may train to lose body weight, others to reverse diabetes, while others may focus on physical appearance.

Perhaps the most significant reason most people start exercising is to lose body weight and improve their aesthetic appearance. However, some health experts think people focus too much on weight loss and forget about the numerous health benefits of regular exercise.

The primary aim of engaging in regular physical training must be improving health, especially metabolic health, as good metabolic health will result in an increased feeling of well-being and improved looks.

Aerobic and Cardio

When it comes to exercise choices, aerobic exercise is the most common choice, and there is a reason for that. If you look at the list of the most common causes of mortality in the US, you can see that people are most likely to die early due to poor heart or respiratory health.

Aerobic exercise is sometimes called cardio. For example, bodybuilders prefer using the term cardio, whereas women going to weight loss classes are more likely to use the term aerobic. However, it is important to know that both terms can be used interchangeably, as they indicate a similar type of exercise.

Before discussing this exercise type further, it is worth understanding that it would be even better to call these exercises a "cardiorespiratory workout" since they are equally good for cardiorespiratory health. That is why we said that aerobic exercise is one of the best forms of exercise for reducing the risk of mortality and disability and improving quality of life.

Why is it called aerobic? The term means training with moderate intensity and training "with oxygen." Extensive training results in so-called anaerobic respiration, which is not the right and efficient way to burn calories. Extensive training will not necessarily result in more significant weight loss or better cardiorespiratory health. [10]

Hence, most experts recommend that one should engage in thirty to sixty minutes of moderate-intensity aerobic exercise at least five days a week. One may even do these exercises daily.[11]

Since aerobic exercise is more beneficial when done with moderate intensity, it is suitable for most of the population.

There are many types of aerobic exercises, like weight loss classes or instructor-led aerobic sessions, cycling, swimming, walking, rowing, elliptical training, running, jumping, and dancing.

Some of the benefits of aerobic exercise are:

- **Excellent cardiovascular conditioning**—thus helping normalize blood pressure and reduce the risk of cardiovascular or heart diseases. Better vascular health is also good for preventing stroke.

- **Respiratory conditioning**—aerobic exercise enhances respiratory volume and reduces residual respiratory volume. Those who engage in aerobic exercises are more likely to have healthy lungs. Thus, these exercises may help reduce the risk of severe pulmonary infections too.

- **Better blood flow to the brain**—aerobic training could be considered one of the better ways of staying alert, enhancing brain health, and reducing the risk of age-related mental decline. These benefits occur not just due to enhanced blood flow but also due to many neurochemical changes that take place following aerobic exercise.

- **Better for musculoskeletal health**—aerobic exercises are not the best way to build muscles, but they improve muscle tone and help reduce muscle fat accumulation. This is also one of the most effective ways to reduce the risk of joint disorders. However, if you are living with joint disorders, engaging in low-impact exercises like cycling or swimming is better.

- **Helps reduce blood sugar and bad cholesterol**—among the different forms of exercise, aerobic training is perhaps the most effective way to reduce cholesterol and normalize blood sugar. After all, it is about burning many calories in a short time.

- **Weight loss**—most weight loss programs use aerobic training as, again, nothing is better for burning many calories in a short time than aerobic training.

- **Good for mental health**—one of the less-often discussed benefits of this exercise form. However, most would agree that nothing is better for mental health than a morning walk, jogging, or swimming. Most aerobic activities are quite interesting. Additionally, it seems that aerobic training helps alter neural connections and energy supply pathways, thus boosting mental health. It also helps reduce stress hormone levels.

One of the important factors to consider when engaging in aerobic training is exercise intensity. There are many ways of monitoring exercise intensity, including gut feeling and monitoring respiratory rate or even fatigue level.

However, the most dependable way to calculate exercise intensity is by monitoring heart rate and doing some basic mathematics. This will provide more precise information about exercise intensity.

Not only that, but it will also help you understand some of the essential concepts before starting any workout or training.

First and foremost, calculate your maximum heart rate. Your heart should not beat for long above these numbers; otherwise, exercise may pose a health risk. Your maximum heart rate depends on your age, and it is pretty simple to calculate: just subtract your age from 220. So if your age is forty, the maximum number of times your heart should beat is not more than 180 times per minute (220 – 40 = 180 beats per minute [bpm]).[12]

Once you know the maximum permissible heart rate for your age, next calculate your **heart rate reserve (HRR).** For this, you need to know your average resting rate, which is generally between seventy and eighty beats per minute. If you have a health band or other wearable, this will make it easier to learn your average resting heart rate. To calculate HRR, subtract your average resting heart rate from your maximum heart rate. Thus, for example, if you have a resting heart rate of seventy bpm and your age is forty, then your HRR is 180 – 70 = 110 bpm.

Most experts agree that moderate exercise makes the heart work at 50 to 70 percent of its level. This level of exertion is optimal for strengthening the heart muscle without overburdening it, effectively enhancing cardiovascular health and endurance. Hence, assuming an HRR of 110, you would multiply that number by 0.5 or 0.7 to calculate your intensity zone. Thus, 50 percent of the intensity would be your resting heart rate (70 bpm) + (110 x 0.5), which is 125 bpm. So, if your target is 50 percent exercise intensity, your heart rate must be around 125 or a bit higher when doing aerobic exercise.

After addressing your cardiovascular and respiratory health, which can enhance metabolic health and reduce fatigue during physical activities, it's a good idea to consider building lean muscle mass, increasing strength, and improving endurance. The most effective way to achieve these goals is through strength training.

One of the questions that many people ask is whether they can combine multiple types of workouts. The answer is yes. It is usually even better to combine different kinds of exercises. Indeed, building muscle mass helps increase the benefits of aerobic training. Similarly, those engaged in strength training would benefit from a cardio workout, which should be a part of their regular training.

Hence, it would be unwise to see different exercise types as entirely different. On the contrary, they often complement each other's health benefits. Combining multiple types of exercise produces optimal health and the best results.

Strength and Resistance Training

Strength training is about lifting weights and using dumbbells, bar-bells, kettlebells, and various resistance training machines installed at gyms. Although there are many modes of resistance training, it is worth understanding that one does not necessarily need a great deal of equipment to carry out these kinds of exercises.

There is no scientific proof that such equipment enables one to gain muscle mass, strength, and endurance. For most people, a couple of dumbbells suffices. One can even do resistance training with resistance bands. If you dislike using equipment, no problem—you can use body weight for resistance training.

There are many reasons why resistance training is important for everyone. Unfortunately, many people looking to lose weight tend to neglect resistant training. Similarly, older adults are more likely to go for a brisk walk than engage in resistance training. However, strength or resistance training is necessary for all due to its unique health benefits.

Many overweight individuals complain that they cannot lose much body weight despite regularly attending their aerobic classes and following dietary recommendations. However, these individuals do not realize that their efforts do not provide sufficient results due to insufficient muscle mass.

It is simple to understand that muscles burn calories; fat tissues do not burn calories when one is exercising. This means that the greater one's muscle mass, the more calories one can burn in a given time. It is quite like an automobile: one with a larger engine burns more fuel.

If you are among those struggling to lose body weight despite regular aerobic training, it is quite possible that you have low muscle mass and, thus, a low metabolic rate.

Additionally, strength training can significantly boost *resting metabolic rate.* Do this simple experiment: train with some really heavy weights for forty-five minutes, and you will notice that it may take your heart rate several hours to return to its preworkout level.

Similarly, in older adults, one of the biggest problems is fat accumulation in muscles and muscle degeneration. And strength training can reverse many of these changes caused by aging and a sedentary lifestyle.

Needless to say, toned muscles improve body shape and look good. However, one must realize that muscles also play a vital role in many metabolic activities. For example, muscles consume much glucose-stored energy, and higher muscle mass can ensure low insulin resistance.

Although everyone understands that weight training helps build muscle strength and endurance, many do not realize that physical training is also suitable for bone health. Most people visualize bone as something inert that just supports your body. However, that is untrue—bones are highly dynamic. Remember that all your red blood cells and immune cells are produced by your bones (bone marrow). In addition, bones are the most abundant source of stem cells and thus play a vital role in body regeneration.

Bones are continually remodeled. Two different types of bone cells play an important role in bone remodeling. One type of cell removes unnecessary bony structures, and the other type creates new bone cells. Strength training can considerably strengthen your bones, along with skeletal muscles. People just neglect the role of resistance training in strengthening bones, as unlike changes in muscle, changes in bone mass are not visible to the naked eye.

Healthy lean mass is also vital to heart health. After all, a considerable number of blood vessels are in skeletal muscles. Therefore, training your muscles and increasing their mass can significantly boost vascular health. These actions also send positive signals to various organs and may have wide-ranging health benefits.

So, next time you pick up a barbell or dumbbell, remember that pumping iron is not just about building muscle mass. It has many other health effects. For example, higher levels of lean mass result in an easier time burning fat, create better metabolic health, increase metabolic rate, reduce insulin resistance, and more.

To sum up, strength training is all about:[13]

- Greater muscle mass
- Greater muscle strength and endurance
- Better body shape
- Ability to burn more calories in fewer minutes of training
- Higher metabolic rate
- Ability to burn more fat in less time
- Improved metabolic health
- Antiaging effects
- Greater bone mass and aiding in the prevention of age-related weakening of bones

HIIT

Aerobic and strength training are the two most common and basic kinds of exercise everyone must engage in. However, other exercise types may be a better choice in specific circumstances. High-intensity interval training (HIIT), for example, is an exercise type that might be better for boosting metabolism and getting results in a shorter period of time.

One of the issues many people face these days is that they do not have sufficient time for exercise. And HIIT, in many cases, provides results similar to aerobic training but in less time.

Here, it is vital to understand that HIIT is not a replacement for aerobic training. On the contrary, as the name of this exercise suggests, it causes more significant stress on the cardiorespiratory system in a much shorter time frame.

This means HIIT may adversely affect those living with suboptimal cardiac health. It may not be a good choice for those with poor health, older adults, and those with joint disorders. Nonetheless, it is a good choice for busy individuals who constantly complain about lack of time. Many people gain excellent results by only dedicating fifteen to twenty minutes to HIIT.

So, what is HIIT? In this exercise form, one alternates short bursts of high-intensity exercise with low-intensity recovery periods. For example, one may sprint for three minutes, then walk briskly for another five minutes.

Unlike aerobic exercises that are done at moderate intensity and for a long time, these short bursts of high intensity cause a great deal of stress on the heart and other body systems.

However, this exercise has some distinct benefits. It is excellent for boosting metabolism for a long period of time. Further, one can achieve excellent results in a short period of time. For many people, it may produce results in a much shorter time frame than regular aerobic training.

One can choose any kind of body weight exercise for this type of training, like sprinting, biking or rope jumping. Most of these exercises can also be done as a part of aerobic training. However, in HIIT, again, one does these exercises for a much shorter time but at a much higher intensity.

This combination of a high-intensity and a low-intensity work-out creates a so-called round or repetition (rep). One might engage in four to six reps/rounds in each training session.

Some of the distinct benefits of HIIT are:[14]

- **Helps burn many calories in a short time:** This is the number-one reason to consider this exercise form. A burst of high-intensity exercise can elevate heart rate and metabolism. That means that one can burn a massive amount of calories in a much shorter time compared to other exercise forms.

- **Elevates metabolic rate for several hours:** One of the secret elements of effective weight loss is elevating one's resting metabolic rate. Studies show that HIIT may result in an elevated heart rate for several hours after the workout. Hence, it can significantly increase one's resting metabolic rate. This kind of effect does not occur with moderate-intensity aerobic workouts like jogging.

- **Helps with losing fat:** Increased energy burning in a short time and elevated metabolic activity results in faster depletion of glucose stores. The body is then forced to mobilize fat stores. Hence, HIIT is one of the most effective forms of exercise for speedier weight loss.

- **Helps with gaining muscle mass:** Although weight training remains the gold standard for building muscles, some people do not seem to benefit from resistance training. Therefore, HIIT may help with gaining muscle mass in some cases.

- **Can improve endurance:** Your endurance or stamina significantly depends on oxygen supply and its consumption by the muscles. Aerobic exercises are pretty good for stamina building. However, HIIT may be a quicker way to achieve high endurance. On the other hand, HIIT is quite good for boosting cardiorespiratory health and improving muscle oxygen consumption.

- **Good for heart health:** HIIT causes significant stress on the cardiovascular system in a short time. Hence, it can considerably increase cardiac reserves; it is suitable for reducing blood pressure and may also help reduce heart rate. That said, as already said, HIIT is not for those living with a weak heart or cardiovascular ailments.

- **Good for metabolic health:** These short bursts of high intensity are quite good for lowering blood sugar for a long time and reducing insulin resistance. Many people living with conditions like obesity and diabetes do not seem to benefit from aerobic training. It seems that HIIT may be a better choice for such people.

- **Improvement to both aerobic and anaerobic performance:** A high-intensity workout followed by a recovery period means that during this workout, the body remains in both aerobic and anaerobic zones. Thus, HIIT is an excellent way to boost aerobic and anaerobic capacity.

It is true that aerobic and weight training are beneficial in most cases, and they are the most commonly recommended exercise forms. However, not all people may get the desired results from those exercises. Some have insufficient time; others just fail to lose body weight through aerobic training.

HIIT may be the right choice of exercise in many instances. It is an even more natural form of physical activity as the human body is made to tolerate short bursts of high-intensity workouts followed by recovery. Moreover, the recovery period here does not mean rest; it just means lowering the exercise intensity.

Stretching Exercises

This is one of the important exercise types. In fact, most exercise programs start with a warmup that includes stretching exercises, as stretching has many unique benefits.

These kinds of exercises are less intensive and might prove a better fit for a wider range of age groups and physical abilities. For example, some older adults living with cardiovascular and other chronic ailments may benefit more from stretching and balance, and these exercises are safe for that population group.

If we carefully look at some traditional forms of exercises like yoga and tai chi, we find that they involve a good deal of stretching. Stretching is also part of activities like bale dancing and martial arts. There is a reason traditional exercise forms and modern health experts favor frequent stretching of muscles.

One of the good things about stretching is that it is pretty simple to learn, and it is also a low-intensity workout in most cases, though not always. Therefore, one does not need any degree of physical preparedness to start doing these kinds of exercises.

To get started with stretching, one must just identify the muscle groups that require stretching. For example, it seems that prolonged sitting results in the tightening of lower back and hip muscles. Thus, any stretching regime must include exercises that stretch these muscles.

One may carry out stretching independently or combine it with other exercise forms. But, of course, this decision depends on one's health conditions and even age.

There are many ways to do stretching. Some of the common ways are:

- **Static stretching:** In this exercise form, you stretch your target group of muscles to the maximum. It may cause pain, so stop stretching if the pain is too much. Next, hold in the position for ten to thirty seconds, and then relax.

- **Dynamic stretching:** This is more commonly done as a warmup. Here, you stretch your muscles to the maximum, but you do not hold them in that place. Instead, you relax immediately. This kind of stretching is done more like an exercise. In fact, many aerobic exercises are types of dynamic stretching.

- **Active stretching:** In this kind of stretching, one uses the force of other muscles to stretch particular muscles. Sometimes, one even utilizes the help of others in active stretching. This kind of stretching may help improve flexibility faster. That is why many sportspeople use active stretching.

- **Ballistic stretching:** This is a less commonly used type that involves repetitive bouncing to stretch specific muscle groups. However, it may not work for many muscle groups.

- **Myofascial release:** People are quite likely to do this type of stretching at the gym or before and after strength training. In these exercises, one uses a roller or similar kind of device to improve tissue blood flow and flexibility. It may also help reduce muscle pain.

People may engage in many other types of stretching exercises under specific conditions.

Many people avoid stretching as they find it a painful activity. Although some pain is normal while stretching, experts say stretching should not cause severe pain. High-intensity pain is a result of overstretching, something that must be avoided.

It's important not to take cues from belly dancers or martial artists for examples of stretching practices. These individuals engage in extreme stretching routines, which are unnecessary for achieving good overall health. Furthermore, their requirements for flexibility often extend beyond the normal range of motion, and they need to attain this flexibility rapidly, which may not be applicable to the average person's health goals.

When using stretching as an exercise, you do not need to go beyond the normal range of motion and do not need to hurry. Stretching should be an enjoyable activity and should have a refreshing and energizing effect on your body.

Some of the benefits of stretching are:[15]

- **Improved physical performance:** Stretching improves blood flow to your muscles and results in enhanced flexibility, which can help improve physical performance.

- **Reduced risk of injuries:** This is arguably the number-one benefit of stretching. People who sit for long hours in front of a screen develop some unique problems, like contraction and weakening of core muscles. That is why the incidence of lower back pain is rising globally. Stretching helps prevent lower back pain and other kinds of physical injuries. More flexibility also means becoming more active.

- **Improved range of motion of joints:** This is a significant problem among older adults. However, stretching is among the best exercises to prevent and manage joint issues. Remember that joint inflammation causes spasms of adjoining muscles; thus, stretching is a must for those prone to joint problems.

- **Improved blood flow:** This factor may help people train better, yet improved blood flow also has numerous benefits for metabolic health. This is why stretching helps manage many chronic health conditions and is not just about enhanced flexibility.

- **Muscles work more efficiently:** Stretching helps people stay active for longer and train better. In addition, one can use it to warm up before different kinds of exercises.

- **Improved ability to carry out daily activities:** Many everyday activities require a great deal of flexibility. Thus, stretching helps. It also improves the range of motion, which may further help one in carrying out daily activities.

Make stretching a ritual before starting to train at a gym, lifting weights, playing sports, and more.

Sports Training

We can all agree that nothing is more pleasurable than participating in the sports of one's choice. Even more rewarding is frequently winning at said sports.

When people are young, they play a lot and they participate in different sports. However, as we grow up, we stop participating in sports and training.

Going to the gym, lifting weights, or attending aerobic classes may provide some good results. But, let us be honest, those activities do not bring the kind of satisfaction we get from participation in sports. Nothing compares to the joy and happiness of training for and playing your favorite sports.

Although sports training is not a distinct kind of exercise, it is a physically demanding activity and thus can be called a type of exercise.

Many individuals simply dislike weight lifting solely for the purpose of muscle strengthening or performing awkward movements to shed body weight. They find these activities too monotonous to maintain. However, sports training offers a distinct experience, primarily due to the enjoyment it brings. It's the element of fun and engagement that sets sports training apart.

Of course, sports training can be highly demanding, depending on the kind of sports one participates in. It often requires different types of exercises, including stretching, weight lifting, resistance training, and aerobics. However, when doing these different exercises, people know why they are doing them and that they will help them get better at a particular sport they enjoy playing.

One can stick to sports training for much longer. Sports also involve movements that are more natural to humans, like jumping and hitting something.

Some of the unique benefits of sports training are:

- One can stick with it for much longer.
- It is generally more attractive than other forms of exercise.
- It may have more significant mental health benefits and bring greater degrees of satisfaction.
- It often involves doing different kinds of exercises like strength training, cardio, and stretching, and thus may have incredible health benefits in the long run.
- It promotes a healthy lifestyle.

So, for most people, there is nothing like sports training to improve fitness, prevent disease, and save on health insurance. On the other hand, if you like sports like soccer, basketball, tennis, softball, and volleyball, there is nothing like sports training. However, one downside is that sports training may sometimes demand more time and resources.

Yoga and Pilates

Yoga, Pilates, and what some call yogalates are low-impact exercises that share many traits. However, there are some differences between these forms of exercise. For example, yoga stresses relaxation and spirituality, whereas Pilates is more about increasing physical movement and strength.

In yoga, a person sits in a specific pose and then moves on to the next pose. In Pilates, one may also form a specific pose; however, one may also apply some force or resistance for extra benefits.

Yoga and Pilates have transformed significantly over the years, which is why we are mentioning them under a single heading. That said, there are many types of yoga and Pilates, and the type of workout one engages in is often dependent on the instructor.

These exercises do not involve jerky motions, which sets them apart from other exercise forms. They also allow a person to focus on breathing and thoughts and thus have more significant mental health benefits.

These exercises are not just good for strength building but also for improving flexibility, balance, mental health, and even rehabilitation.

Over the years, specialists have honed these exercises for special needs. In fact, unlike other exercise forms, both yoga and Pilates were created to prevent, manage, or even treat disease conditions.

Therefore, these exercises are the right choice for those living with chronic ailments. Of course, these exercises help manage issues like back pain, joint pain, injuries, and arthritis. But they also help manage and treat more severe conditions.

For example, yoga may also help improve sleep and reduce stress and depression. It is good for improving digestion, managing metabolic health issues, and more. In addition, there are specific yoga poses to relieve the pain of various internal organs and stimulate their function. Both yoga and Pilates focus heavily on breathing, too.

These exercises often have a cultlike following, and those who become used to them gain many benefits by sticking with them long enough.

Unlike in other exercise forms, minor ailments are often not contraindications for these exercises. That means that these exercise forms may be better suited for those living with health conditions like frequent backaches and gastrointestinal distress.

These exercises may help build muscle strength, improve flexibility, and result in better balance. However, they do not cause much stress on the heart, making them a better choice for those living with cardiac health issues.

Some of the reasons to consider yogalates are:

- Improves strength and endurance
- Enhances flexibility and balance
- Reduces injury risk
- Helps reduce joint pain and lower back pain
- Good for reducing the risk of chronic ailments and even managing disease conditions
- Helps improve focus and mental health

Before we move on to the next topic, it is worth understanding that workouts like yoga are not just for physical health. Yoga is a whole philosophy. So, how much you benefit from it depends on the extent to which you include yoga into your lifestyle. You can practice it merely as a physical exercise or start exploring its philosophy more deeply.

Exercises for Rehabilitation and Recovery

These are the kinds of exercises that your physiotherapist, sports medicine specialist, or doctor would prescribe to overcome specific health conditions. However, these exercises do not truly fit with the types mentioned above, which mainly prevent disease by considerably boosting physical, metabolic, and mental health.

On the other hand, you engage in rehabilitation and recovery exercises to eliminate ailments, trauma, and painful conditions, as in an exercise program to manage lower back pain or knee arthritis. Such exercises are commonly prescribed when one is recovering from severe trauma like spinal trauma or a femur fracture.

Rehabilitation exercises are also needed to recover from other health issues like stroke and even to improve one's condition after a heart attack.

Unlike other exercise forms, these kinds of exercises are best done under supervision as there is a risk of doing more harm than good.

In conclusion, one can see that there are many different types of exercises. Though we mentioned the most common types here, this list is undoubtedly not complete.

One needs to understand that for good health, it is important to get started with some kind of exercise program. Then, one can progress and build on the achieved results. For example, a person may begin with aerobic exercises for a few months and then add resistance exercises. Or one may combine HIIT with resistance training.

Indeed, the most important thing for building good health is getting started. It is quite challenging to get something moving when it is standing still due to high initial resistance. However, as that thing starts moving, it gains momentum, and then much less effort is needed to keep it going.

Make a firm decision and start doing one kind of exercise, any kind. You can improve the quality of the workout at later stages.

The initial phase will always be difficult due to fatigue and body aches. However, as time passes, your body will get used to the physical stress, and things will become easier.

If one sticks to the exercise for long enough, they also become motivated due to visible results. Therefore, it is vital to include exercise in your lifestyle as an essential element, like food and sleep. One should stop considering exercise as something optional or needed for weight loss.

The initial phase generally lasts for a few months for most individuals. So do not expect that you will get used to exercising in a couple of weeks. In fact, the initial few weeks may be relatively easy; after that point, many become discouraged when they don't experience quick results. As a result, many people discontinue exercising at this critical stage without realizing that had they continued, their lives would have changed forever. So start doing exercise, and forget about giving up on it. Instead, let exercise become an essential element of your life.

Since we know that overcoming that early resistance is the most difficult step, in the next chapter, we look at some tips to help you get started and stay motivated.

END-OF-MODULE-II ACTIVITIES

Self-Assessment: Reflect on your personal health goals and current fitness level. Are you looking to lose weight, build muscle, improve flexibility, or enhance overall health?

_____

_____

_____

_____

_____

_____

_____

_____

_____

_____

_____

_____

Research and Selection: Explore different types of exercises (aerobic, strength/resistance training, HIIT, stretching exercises, sports training, yoga, and Pilates) and choose one that aligns with your goals and interests.

_____

_____

_____

_____

_____

_____

_____

_____

_____

_____

_____

_____

Plan Creation: Develop a weekly exercise plan incorporating your selected exercise type. Ensure it's realistic and fits into your daily routine.

_____

_____

_____

_____

_____

_____

_____

_____

_____

_____

_____

_____

_____

_____

_____

_____

Activity Log: For one week, maintain a log of your exercises. Note the type, duration, and how you feel during and after each session.

_____

_____

_____

_____

_____

_____

_____

_____

_____

_____

_____

_____

_____

_____

Evaluation and Reflection: After a week, review your log. Did the exercise type meet your expectations? How did it impact your mood, energy, and overall well-being? Adjust your plan based on this evaluation.

_____

_____

_____

_____

_____

_____

_____

_____

_____

_____

_____

_____

_____

_____

END-OF-MODULE QUIZ

1. **Question:** What is a key benefit of aerobic exercise?

   A) It primarily builds muscle mass.

   B) It improves cardiovascular and respiratory health.

   C) It has no impact on mental health.

   D) It's only effective for young adults.

2. **Question:** What is the primary focus of strength/resistance training?

   A) Enhancing flexibility

   B) Building muscle strength and endurance

   C) Improving cardiovascular fitness

   D) Relaxation and mental focus

3. **Question:** How does high-intensity interval training (HIIT) differ from traditional aerobic exercises?

   A) HIIT is less effective in burning calories.

   B) HIIT involves alternating periods of high- and low-intensity exercise.

   C) HIIT is only for professional athletes.

   D) HIIT focuses on long-duration activities.

4. **Question:** True or False: Yoga and Pilates are primarily beneficial for physical health and have little impact on mental well-being.

A) True

B) False

5. **Question:** What is the main purpose of rehabilitation and recovery exercises?

A) To compete in sports

B) To improve aesthetic appearance

C) To recover from injuries or manage specific health conditions

D) To build large muscle groups

ANSWERS

1. B) It improves cardiovascular and respiratory health.

2. B) Building muscle strength and endurance

3. B) HIIT involves alternating periods of high- and low-intensity exercise.

4. B) False

5. C) To recover from injuries or manage specific health conditions

MODULE III

TIPS FOR GETTING STARTED WITH EXERCISE

Well begun is half done.

—Aristotle

Getting started is the most critical step in achieving anything. Once you have started something, you are already in the game. However, this does not mean that one should rush in, as an ill-planned beginning often results in quitting without achieving anything.

Remember that one cannot move forward by starting and quitting frequently. That is more like one step forward and one back. It is not going to take you anywhere. Therefore, before starting, make a firm decision.

As we have already said, exercise should be an essential part of life, like eating and sleeping. It is time that people stopped viewing it as something elective. Indeed, one needs to develop a habit of exercising regularly. Once it becomes a habit, it starts calling you, like a pang of hunger or the need to sleep.

And remember that just as a person cannot survive without food, one cannot expect to live long without physical activity. Those who do not move enough age quickly, develop many health disorders, and suffer.

Of course, exercise causes pain and fatigue. But this pain and fatigue are controlled. If you do not undergo this controlled pain, you will ultimately experience more severe pain in the form of failing health. Lack of exercise will make your body so weak that you will readily get fatigued.

Thus, pain and fatigue caused by physical training ultimately have a positive effect as they increase your energy reserves. Exercise recharges your body.

So, do not waste time procrastinating. There is no tomorrow. We live today. Dreaming is good, planning is better, and execution is much better. We all know that very few people achieve their New Year's resolutions. Hence, if you want to get fit, remember that action is the key. And there is no better day than today to start taking action.

Of course, you may wonder how to get started, make a plan, and execute it. There are no perfect plans. Moreover, plans are no good without execution. Nonetheless, it is good to have a basic plan to get better results.

So here are some of the essential elements of any exercise plan. Of course, your exercise plan may look different and not have all these elements, but most physical training plans will look similar to this.

Assess Your Fitness Level

To begin with, you need to know who you are and what you are capable of, as this will help you monitor the transformation that will happen.

Unfortunately, many people remain unsatisfied with their results merely because they never assessed their initial fitness level. Thus, they do not have a point of comparison.

There are many things you need to know before starting. However, most of these baseline recordings can be readily done without much expertise.

Start with your body weight and BMI. Of course, calculating BMI requires you to know your height, too. Here, we are not going to discuss what BMI is or how to calculate it as one can readily google it. In addition, many online calculators can help. But remember that body weight and BMI are essential things that anyone should know.

Next, start taking some more complex measurements, like waist circumference. If you are looking to build muscles, you may need to take more detailed body measurements like thigh, biceps, and chest circumference.

These days, smart weighing scales do not cost much. A digital weight scale is a must for every household. It is preferable to invest in one that also provides readings of body composition. Such scales can accurately calculate BMI. However, be careful when interpreting other readings like total fat and muscle mass, as no machine can provide an accurate reading. Those are just rough indicators. Still, knowing these things is worth it.

Once you have basic body readings, it is time to learn your fitness score. You can do some simple tests, like how long it takes you to run one-and-a-half miles if you can run that far. You can also note the number of push-ups you can do in a single go.

These are very basic fitness measurements. However, when you start training, you will be happy to see how much you have changed in just a few months. Depending on the type of exercise you choose, you might be able to easily do twice as many push-ups or run much faster within just three months.

Noting down these basic health and fitness parameters is essential. However, we strongly recommend going further, especially if you have never exercised, have health issues, and are above the age of thirty.

For those who are starting to exercise for the first time and are above the age of thirty, it may be a good idea to get a blood pressure reading. Data suggest that about one-third of adults are either hypertensive or borderline hypertensive. This is important to know before starting any workout plan. Knowing this information helps tailor exercise intensity and type to avoid potential health risks and maximize benefits.

Our next pro tip is to get tested for blood glucose levels. However, instead of fasting blood glucose, go for an HbA1c test that measures the average blood sugar level for the last three months.

If you feel fatigued most of the time, then you should consult your doctor before starting any exercise. In addition, it is generally a good idea to have a complete lab checkup that includes an assessment of liver function and thyroid function and provides some information about nutritional levels of serum calcium, vitamin D, vitamin B12, hemoglobin, and more.

You don't have to go through extensive testing to check all those parameters. Most labs provide different kinds of panels, and getting tested for these things is pretty simple. However, having a deeper understanding of your health can significantly improve the effectiveness of your exercise program.

For example, low thyroid function may make any physical training ineffective. Similarly, low calcium and vitamin D levels may prevent one from making expected gains. However, most of these conditions are readily managed if the person is aware of their condition.

Once you know all about your fitness levels, start designing your fitness program.

Create Your Fitness Program

Setting your fitness goals shouldn't be an overwhelming task. In fact, tailoring your fitness plan to your goals is often the best approach, as you're the best judge of the changes you want to achieve. Start by asking yourself a fundamental question: **What do I want to accomplish?** Your fitness goal might be to lose weight, run a 10K, build muscle, or complete a marathon.

The key is to set goals that are realistic and attainable. For instance, while not everyone may be ready to tackle a marathon, setting a target to run a 5K in under thirty minutes is both challenging and achievable. Remember, your fitness journey is unique to you. Choose goals that inspire you and are aligned with your personal aspirations and abilities.

When setting goals, remember that health is more important than your looks or what you achieve in the next twelve months. For example, running a marathon is not essentially a healthy activity. Similarly, building massive muscles like a bodybuilder's does not mean good health.

Therefore, our recommendation is to go for a **balanced routine**. This means building a beach-ready body without massive mass gain, trying to run 5K, improving your energy levels, boosting cardiorespiratory health, becoming more active, and so on.

Of course, start with something more realistic, like 150 minutes of aerobic exercise per week, and start with moderate intensity, something like 50 percent intensity. You can increase the intensity level after a few months. However, your ultimate goal should be 300 minutes of exercise weekly. If you are short on time, HIIT may be the right choice. If you hate working out, think of joining a tennis club or engaging in a similar kind of demanding aerobic activity that is more interesting for you.

To optimize your fitness routine, it's beneficial to diversify your exercises. A balanced approach that includes both aerobic workouts and resistance training can enhance overall fitness.

For those focusing on improving endurance, aim for exercises with lower resistance and higher repetitions. This method helps build stamina and cardiovascular health. On the other hand, if your goal is to gain muscle mass, focus on performing fewer repetitions with heavier weights. This strategy targets muscle growth and strength development.

Our aim here is to give a general idea of how your exercise program should look. Of course, this book is not about designing an exercise program. Instead, we want to explain some of the important underlying principles and provide you with the right mindset to start thinking in the right direction. When it comes to designing a fitness program, there are many apps and online resources that can guide you well.

The next thing to remember is not to overstress from day one. **Start slowly, and keep progressing**. Many people stress out too much in the initial phase. This may cause injuries, severe body aches, and even serious health issues. Do not listen to anyone in this matter; just listen to your body.

Of course, you must go through some pain, and any workout program must be moderately challenging, or you won't progress. But we suggest avoiding overenthusiasm. Remember that if you stick to your plans for long enough, you will make progress, but if you have to quit, then all is lost.

Making the workout your habit is essential, and it should be a **part of your daily routine**. Therefore, also focus on making your exercise program enjoyable. Training for a few weeks is one thing, but sticking to it for months or years is different. Thus, include **variety** in your exercise program too.

For example, perhaps you train intensively with weights for a few months before summer. However, during summer, you might focus less on weight training and more on jogging, swimming, and other outdoor activities.

If you train for five days per week in a gym in winter, you may reduce it to three in summer, and during those warm days, you can focus more on building stamina or endurance.

Also, do not forget about sufficient rest. Here again, listen to your body; it does not matter what self-proclaimed health experts or websites recommend. There is nothing worse than a burnout effect. On the other hand, constant pain might be discouraging. So, if you cannot train five days a week, three or four days are also fine until you progress and stop feeling fatigued. Persistence is the key to success here.

Before we move on to the next tip, here is one more piece of pro advice: When planning physical activities, also plan your diet, which may include supplementation. The right kind of diet and health supplements can do wonders, and they can enhance your results.

Invest in Equipment and a New Lifestyle

To make your whole experience pleasurable, make fitness your life-style. This will not only improve results; it will also motivate you significantly. This may even mean changing your wardrobe. For example, it may mean less focus on formal wear and more on sports styles. Thus, invest in good running shoes, wearables, different types of equipment, smart tracking devices, and more.

Remember that investing extends beyond exercise equipment, as that is the bare minimum. Invest in things that bring you pleasure and help you keep motivated. For example, ear pods do not have much to do with exercise, but listening to hi-fi music can make jogging much more enjoyable.

Get Started

Now you know what it takes to get started, have developed the right mindset plan, and have invested in some gear. It is time to start training now. This is ultimately the most important thing. All the preparation was done to get started in the right way.

When exercising, start slowly and do not forget to warm up. Many people are injured due to insufficient warmup. A good warmup routine must include light exercises and some stretching. This is especially true for older adults, who are more prone to injuries.

When starting an exercise program, it is a good idea not to do everything in a single session as that may be very tiring. For example, you might jog in the morning and do strength training in the evening. Or even better, do yoga in the evening.

Remember that although you have made a plan and must stick to it to the greatest degree possible, you can still make exceptions and changes to that initial plan. After all, when planning, you might underestimate or overestimate your physical capabilities. Thus, as you continue with your exercise program, tweaking and fine-tuning are essential elements. However, by doing so, you are not breaking any law.

For example, when you start exercising, you may realize that something is not fitting into your lifestyle. You may prefer hanging out with friends on Saturday evenings. Thus, light morning training on that day might be a better option for you. Do not overstress yourself, as exercising has to be an enjoyable activity.

Keep Monitoring

Keeping track of your progress is a crucial and motivating aspect of any training regimen. However, it's important to approach this with moderation. For instance, if you're exercising for weight loss, resist the temptation to weigh yourself daily. This frequent monitoring can be misleading and unnecessary. Instead, opt for a monthly check-in to assess your progress.

The rationale behind less frequent monitoring is simple. Significant weight loss doesn't happen overnight, and your weight can fluctuate throughout the day due to factors like hydration levels and food intake. Giving yourself time between checks allows for a more accurate and encouraging reflection of your hard work and progress.

Similarly, suppose someone starts exercising to gain muscle mass. In that case, one may not experience much change initially, as the body slowly starts replacing fats accumulated below the skin and even in muscle cells with muscle fibers.

Additionally, remember that it is absolutely normal to change goals. Let's say that initially, you set out to lose ten pounds a month. That may be a too-ambitious target. You can later revise it to seven pounds after monitoring. Realistic goals and achieving them help you stay motivated.

You should not monitor physical parameters only. Assess other elements like your motivation level and exercise regularity over time. These things are even more important to monitor. For example, if you feel demotivated, using health coach services may help you stay motivated.

The Triangle of Success

Exercising is good, but it is not enough to produce sufficient results. Therefore, although this book focuses mainly on exercise and its benefits, that does not mean one should not consider other lifestyle measures.

One of the most effective ways to meet your goals is to remember the triangle of success when exercising. One side of this triangle is your exercise plan. However, the other two sides, dietary measures, and supplements, also play an equal role in the success of any exercise regime.

Always ensure that you carry out specific dietary measures along with exercise. For example, most medium-size chocolate bars contain 400 to 600 calories. During a one-hour workout, one may barely burn 400 to 600 calories, pointing to the fact that a weight loss program might not work without dietary measures.

Of course, remember that exercise is still beneficial for health even if you do not experience weight loss.

Similarly, those building muscles need massive amounts of proteins and various micronutrients. For example, a 160-pound man may need almost 150 grams of protein daily to build muscles fast. He would also need a lot of energy supply, vitamins, minerals, fatty acids, and other nutrients.

There is indeed nothing like a well-planned diet. However, we do not recommend dieting as it increases the risk of malnutrition. Prolonged dieting may cause deficiencies of various micronutrients and harm health in many ways. So do not confuse dietary planning with dieting. Dietary planning means counting calories, ensuring an ample supply of vital nutrients, avoiding poor-quality nutrients, and more.

Along with diet, dietary supplements may also help improve results. Here again, we are not recommending any specific health supplement. Instead, we are suggesting that if you are living with specific nutritional deficiencies, they might ultimately become your bottleneck. For example, many people live with low vitamin D levels or consume insufficient amounts of omega-3 fatty acids. Thus, supplementing your diet with specific supplements may be the right idea. However, the choice of supplement depends on your health status.

Just be warned that there is no magic pill in the world. There is no substitute for exercise. So keep in mind that first, you should start exercising. At the same time, you should start making dietary changes and eating healthy foods—high-protein foods, fruits, and veggies. If needed, add a couple of supplements to your diet plan to enhance your results.

Keep Learning and Improving Your Technique

When you start exercising, you will realize that taking care of your health requires a great deal of learning. You will have to keep learning new exercises, understanding how to do them properly, and how to prevent injuries. You might even consult coaches and sports medicine specialists from time to time to enhance their knowledge.

As you progress in your fitness journey, undoubtedly, a multitude of questions will arise. These might include inquiries about the correct way to perform push-ups, determining the optimal number of reps, managing rest periods between different exercises, and establishing the frequency of breaks.

What makes these things complicated is that there are no right or wrong answers to many of these questions. Many things are individual. Some may benefit from more reps and less resistance, while others may benefit from a low rep count.

So, we hope our tips will help you get started on your journey to good health. Remember that it is important to understand underlying principles, plan your journey, and then get started and stick to your plans, albeit with some changes.

In the next chapter, we will look at ways exercise can help you regulate your appetite, help with weight loss, and more.

To repeat, weight loss is not the sole purpose of physical training, but it is one of the important aims, considering that many people in the developed world are overweight and addicted to food.

END-OF-MODULE-III ACTIVITIES

Explore Your Fitness Path

Self-Assessment: Reflect on your current fitness level and health. Are you just starting, steadily improving, or already at an advanced stage? Identify your primary health goals.

_____

_____

_____

_____

_____

_____

_____

_____

_____

_____

_____

_____

Personalized Exercise Plan: Develop a weekly exercise schedule tailored to your fitness level and objectives. This plan should include a mix of cardiovascular, strength, and flexibility exercises. Ensure the plan fits into your daily routine realistically.

_____

_____

_____

_____

_____

_____

_____

_____

_____

_____

_____

_____

_____

Implementation and Observation: Commit to your exercise plan for a week. Observe any changes in your mood, energy, or sleep patterns. How do you feel physically and mentally after each exercise session?

_____

_____

_____

_____

_____

_____

_____

_____

_____

_____

_____

_____

_____

_____

Journaling: Document your daily exercise activities, noting the exercise type, exercise duration, and your thoughts on each session. Track any obstacles you encounter and how you address them.

_____

_____

_____

_____

_____

_____

_____

_____

_____

_____

_____

_____

_____

Reflection and Adjustment: After a week, review your exercise journal. What aspects of your plan were successful, and which areas need improvement? Adjust your exercise plan accordingly for the upcoming week.

_____

_____

_____

_____

_____

_____

_____

_____

_____

_____

_____

_____

_____

END-OF-MODULE QUIZ

1. **Question:** What is the benefit of incorporating a variety of exercises into your routine?

   A) It enhances only cardiovascular health.

   B) It reduces the effectiveness of the workout.

   C) It helps in targeting different muscle groups and improves overall fitness.

   D) It only improves flexibility.

2. **Question:** Why is it important to gradually increase the intensity and duration of your workouts?

   A) To reduce the risk of injury

   B) To make the workout easier

   C) It has no impact on the workout

   D) To decrease overall fitness levels

3. **Question:** What is the significance of keeping an exercise journal?

   A) It is only for professional athletes.

   B) It helps track progress and identify areas for improvement.

   C) It has no real purpose.

   D) It should be done only if instructed by a doctor.

4. Question: True or False: Adjusting your fitness plan over time is a sign of failure.

A) True

B) False

5. Question: What role does self-assessment play in your fitness journey?

A) It's unnecessary and can be skipped.

B) It helps in setting unrealistic fitness goals.

C) It's crucial for understanding your starting point and measuring progress.

D) It only helps in choosing the right exercise equipment.

ANSWERS

1. C) It helps in targeting different muscle groups and improves overall fitness.

2. A) To reduce the risk of injury

3. B) It helps track progress and identify areas for improvement.

4. B) False

5. C) It's crucial for understanding your starting point and measuring progress.

MODULE IV

HOW EXERCISE HELPS CURB APPETITE

P eople often exercise to reduce body weight and improve physi-cal and mental health. Everyone who exercises would agree that it affects mood and appetite. However, there are conflicting theories and findings regarding the effect of exercise on appetite.

It is logical to believe that if you burn calories, the body will likely ask for more food to compensate for the loss. This is partially true. However, appetite regulation occurs in a more complex way.

Of course, most people feel an increased urge to eat food after some physical exertion. However, have you noticed that this only occurs after short periods of physical activity? If you exercise for a long time, it does not truly increase your appetite. In fact, after prolonged exercise, you may feel fatigued and have a reduced urge to eat.

It seems that there is more than one way in which exercise affects appetite. However, if you do the right kind of exercise, it can help curb appetite and reduce obesity.

There are approximately fifteen to twenty major hormones that can influence appetite. For example, gut hormones play the most crucial role in appetite regulation, at least in the short- and mid-term. If you have a heavy meal, they immediately send a signal to the brain to stop eating.

However, the gut is not the only organ with a say in how many calories you consume. For example, if you are in a bad mood, you might not want to have food. On the other hand, some people affected by anxiety or depression may engage in binge eating. For them, food is like a medicine that helps them overcome stress. But binge eating is bad medicine, causing more harm than good.

So, we need to understand that appetite control is a complex mechanism. Along with the gut, brain, muscles, and even fat tissues help regulate appetite. In addition, exercise can modulate the activity of different body tissues and organs and thus help curb hunger. That said, the long-term influence of exercise is mild and may vary.

The two most significant hormones known to regulate appetite and energy supplies are **ghrelin** and **leptin**. [16]

Ghrelin increases appetite, whereas leptin helps curb appetite. Thus, these hormones have an opposing action, and exercise can affect their secretion and influence their appetite.

Although ghrelin and leptin have opposing actions, they also differ in many other ways. For example, studies suggest that ghrelin is a short-acting hormone, whereas leptin starts acting relatively slowly and has a longer-lasting action.

Studies show that a slight upsurge in energy requirement caused by stress or short and extensive physical activity may cause an increase in ghrelin and may stimulate appetite. This is logically a compensatory mechanism.

However, as noted above, most people who exercise have noticed that prolonged physical training does not increase appetite and may help curb the excessive desire to eat food. Studies suggest that prolonged activity does not cause an increase in ghrelin and may have a role in boosting the body's leptin supply.

Thus, five to ten minutes of extensive training would not curb your appetite; however, if you train for longer, like thirty minutes or more, you will curb your appetite. Shorter exercise sessions will not increase ghrelin, boost leptin supply, or increase other gut hormones like PYY, GLP-1, and PP, which are potent appetite regulators.[17]

Moreover, it is worth noting that all kinds of exercises help regulate appetite in the long run. For example, in some, an acute bout of physical exertion may increase ghrelin a bit. However, this is a short-lasting hormone. In the long run, exercise instead increases leptin a bit, curbing appetite and thus helping with weight loss.

Interestingly, when it comes to the effect of exercise on leptin (appetite-suppressing hormone) levels, it appears that exercise can both reduce and increase levels of this hormone. Studies show that short-term physical exertion does not curb appetite as it not only increases ghrelin (for a short period) but also reduces leptin.

Similarly, studies show that the body will reduce leptin levels if you train too extensively, but it will not essentially boost ghrelin levels. In this case, reduced leptin results in increased appetite. For most people, training too extensively, resulting in a calorie expenditure of more than 800 kcal, may reduce circulating leptin levels.

So, when one is exercising for weight loss or to counter obesity, these things are necessary to understand. If you feel that exercise increases your appetite, you might not be training effectively and sufficiently. You are expending too little energy and training too little.

However, this does not mean you should start running for an hour to curb your appetite. Running for an hour would help burn many calories. But it would also stimulate appetite.

Indeed, to curb appetite, you need to find that golden line. This means you should train for a long time and engage in moderate-intensity exercise to curb hunger. An aerobic session or resistance training for thirty to sixty minutes a day will curb appetite. However, if you overdo it, the final effect may be quite the opposite.

This may also explain why some people who train extensively for weight loss fail to achieve results. In most instances, people are just not training sufficiently, not burning enough calories, and yet stimulating their appetite. Yet in a few cases, individuals become overenthusiastic and start training too extensively.

Body weight or fat has accumulated over a period of years. It occurs due to a sedentary lifestyle and consuming high-calorie foods. No one should expect the changes that have happened in the body due to years of neglect to be reversed in a few weeks. However, if you train with moderate intensity and stick with it for long enough, you are bound to experience results.

Understanding ghrelin and leptin and their role in modulating appetite is essential. However, it is equally vital to understand how exercise affects these two crucial hormones that modulate appetite.

It would be unwise to think this is the only way to control appetite. In the human body, every function is maintained in very complex ways. Think of the heart, for example. Its activity can be regulated by hormones, fluid and electrolyte balance, nutrients, the autonomous nervous system, and more.

Thus, there are many ways in which the body regulates appetite. Accordingly, there are multiple ways of understanding the energy requirement of various body parts. Certain mechanisms sometimes stimulate or curb hunger for a short time, while other agents may have long-term effects.

Just look at the findings that suggest that even changes in body temperature due to exercise can alter appetite. As you train harder, your body temperature rises a bit. This can have a tremendous impact on appetite and metabolism.

Even a minute increase in body temperature due to prolonged physical activity can stimulate sensory receptors (TRPV1 receptors) and curb appetite. This explains why people with fever dislike eating so much.[18]

This increase in body temperature can also result in increased metabolic activity and mobilization of fat stores. In addition, some new findings suggest that certain herbs, supplements, or foods work by modulating TRPV1 receptors and promoting weight loss (like capsaicin). Thus, they are rightly called fat burners or supplements inducing thermogenesis.

Exercise can also influence the working of various organs. For example, the human gut has a significant say in appetite for obvious reasons. It is worth understanding that exercise also affects gut functioning. For example, exercise can increase PYY, GLP-1, and PP levels, as we have seen, thus causing so-called exercise-induced anorexia.

How exercise affects appetite has remained a neglected subject, and doctors still have a limited understanding of its mechanism. However, as the prevalence of obesity and metabolic disorders increases, researchers are also becoming increasingly interested in how exercise can be used as a tool to curb appetite.

Just consider a new finding regarding the role of lactic acid. Health experts have mostly viewed lactic acid as a metabolic waste that causes muscle soreness and fatigue and must be removed from the body. However, new studies show that it is a potent signaling molecule.[19]

This means that lactic acid levels in the body can influence metabolic rate and even appetite. This is because the body keeps sensing every minute change within it, and it keeps track of lactic acid. Experts have found that lactic acid reduces energy intake. It is another indicator that moderate-intensity exercise is essential to curb appetite.

Every organ in the body is interconnected. Thus, exercise-associated changes in one organ affect the working of others. Exercise not only influences appetite or total calorie intake but may even influence your preference for certain foods in the long run.

Therefore, biochemical changes in the body are not the only way exercise affects your appetite. If you exercise and spend time training, you are less likely to develop chronic stress, anxiety, depression, and other mental health issues. You are also less likely to abuse alcohol and street drugs. This would also modulate your appetite and help normalize your total calorie intake.

Thus, it is also vital to understand that exercising improves mental health and can help curb appetite in this way. It is no secret that many people try to overcome mental health issues through binge eating. They almost become addicted to food. Replace your food addiction with exercise to get metabolically and even mentally healthy.

Changes in mood and the brain gradually occur if you continue to exercise regularly. Consequently, most people who stick to their exercise plan for six months or more notice a significant change in their mood and even thought patterns, as well as see a change in their relation to food.

Exercise will change your body composition, and this will alter your hormonal health. For example, you will have fewer *adipokines* (bioactive peptides produced by adipose tissue, involved in metabolic regulation and inflammation) and less inflammation. This may also translate into a change in appetite.

When we talk about curbing appetite, we are not just referring to changes in total calorie intake. It is also about qualitative changes. As we mentioned above, exercise will start influencing your food choices.

We have all seen images of physically fit people who exercise regularly. And in these images, we see the subjects eating healthy foods like lots of green veggies and high-quality proteins, not fries and soda.

These changes in food consumption are both conscious and unconscious. Of course, once you start exercising, you will naturally begin to focus on a healthy diet, start making healthy choices, and avoid calorie-packed processed foods.

However, what is interesting to note is that many such changes come naturally. For example, those who exercise for a long time see that their food preferences change, in many cases, without making any significant effort.

Once you have experienced and become addicted to endorphins released by physical training, you are less likely to seek pleasure in certain foods. But, regretfully, most unhealthy foods are also addictive. Exercise can help overcome that addiction.

People who train physically are less likely to engage in binge eating and more likely to make healthy food choices consciously and unconsciously. For example, if you exercise regularly for months or years, you will note that you have developed an appetite for fruits, veggies, fresh fruit juices, and more. At the same time, you will note you have started disliking fried items, processed foods, alcohol, and more.

So when you exercise, you are not just burning calories, mobilizing fats, and building muscles. It influences every body part, from toe to head.

The health benefits of exercise are multidimensional. It helps to move from a fatter to a flatter tummy and to build strong muscles. It also causes biochemical changes in the body, modulating your hormones, immunity, and various signaling molecule levels. Further, it modifies your brain function and has a broad impact on your psychology.

Of course, remember that everything is good in moderation, and this is also true for exercise. However, if you overdo it, it may even harm your health. Learn to listen to your body and follow the middle golden line when exercising. You need time and experience to understand these things and develop the ability to listen to what your body is trying to tell you.

Exercise means millions of large and small changes in your body. To keep you motivated, we will look at some of the better-known benefits of exercise. Nearly all of those who exercise can expect to experience these benefits to a greater or lesser degree and thus save on health insurance.

END-OF-MODULE-IV ACTIVITIES

Balancing Appetite through Exercise

Appetite Awareness: Reflect on how your current exercise habits influence your appetite. Do you notice changes in hunger levels after different types of workouts?

_____

_____

_____

_____

_____

_____

_____

_____

_____

_____

_____

_____

Exercise and Eating Log: For one week, keep a detailed log of your exercise sessions alongside your meals. Note the type, duration, and intensity of the exercise, as well as the timing and content of your meals.

_____

_____

_____

_____

_____

_____

_____

_____

_____

_____

_____

_____

_____

Observation and Analysis: Pay close attention to any patterns that emerge between your physical activity and eating habits. Do longer or more intense workouts affect your hunger differently?

_____

_____

_____

_____

_____

_____

_____

_____

_____

_____

_____

_____

_____

_____

Mindful Eating Post-Exercise: After each workout, practice mindful eating. Notice if exercising influences your food choices or portion sizes.

Reflection and Adjustment: After a week, review your exercise and eating log. Identify any connections between exercise and appetite regulation. Consider how you might adjust your exercise routine to better manage your appetite and dietary choices.

_____

_____

_____

_____

_____

_____

_____

_____

_____

_____

_____

_____

END-OF-MODULE QUIZ

1. Question: How does regular exercise typically affect appetite hormones like ghrelin and leptin?

A) Increases ghrelin and decreases leptin

B) Decreases ghrelin and increases leptin

C) No effect on either hormone

D) Increases both ghrelin and leptin

2. Question: What is the effect of short, high-intensity workouts on appetite?

A) They significantly reduce appetite.

B) They have no impact on appetite.

C) They may temporarily increase appetite.

D) They change food preferences toward unhealthy choices.

3. Question: How does prolonged moderate exercise affect hunger?

A) It increases hunger significantly.

B) It has a mild or no effect on hunger.

C) It greatly decreases hunger.

D) It leads to binge eating postexercise.

4. **Question:** True or False: Regular exercise can lead to healthier food choices over time.

A) True

B) False

5. **Question:** What role does mindful eating play in the relationship between exercise and appetite?

A) It has no role.

B) It exacerbates postexercise hunger.

C) It helps recognize and respond to the body's hunger cues more accurately.

D) It increases cravings for high-calorie foods.

ANSWERS

1. B) Decreases ghrelin and increases leptin

2. C) They may temporarily increase appetite.

3. B) It has a mild or no effect on hunger.

4. A) True

5. C) It helps recognize and respond to the body's hunger cues more accurately.

MODULE V

BENEFITS OF REGULAR PHYSICAL ACTIVITY

There are millions of reasons to start exercising, and we are here to look at some of the most common health benefits of exercise. But of course, once you start exercising, you will get all these benefits and many more. In fact, after six months of regular exercise, you will feel transformed and as if you are a new person.

So why delay this incredible journey to self-transformation?

Weight Control

Although we've stressed that exercise should encompass more than just weight control, it's undeniable that weight management serves as a significant initial incentive for many individuals to begin exercising. In this context, exercise is considered one of the healthiest approaches to achieving weight loss.

In the Western world, statistics reveal a concerning trend: nearly 40 percent of the population is classified as obese, with an additional 30 percent falling into the overweight category. This alarming data indicates that a significant 70 percent of all adults are in need of weight reduction strategies.[20]

The positive impact of weight loss through exercise is not only a physical transformation but also a powerful source of motivation for those on a fitness journey.

In a paradigm shift within the medical community, obesity is no longer viewed merely as a contributing factor to various health conditions like diabetes and heart disease. Medical professionals and organizations in the US and Europe now recognize obesity as a standalone disease. This reclassification underscores the urgency of treating obesity, positioning weight loss not just as a beneficial strategy but also as a critical treatment approach in its own right.[21]

When starting exercise for weight loss, remember that it works better when used along with dietary measures.

There are two main reasons for obesity: higher calorie intake and low calorie expenditure.

Exercise helps boost metabolism and increase calorie expenditure. However, if you continue filling your body with a great deal of fuel, you might not get satisfactory results or make much progress.

When we speak of dietary measures, we do not mean dieting. Dieting is not the right way to reduce body weight as it increases the risk of nutritional deficiencies and may harm health. Instead, dietary measures mean counting calories and reducing total daily calorie intake.

Of course, exercise is not a magic pill, and it takes really hard work to burn calories. Burning fats is even more difficult. Remember that 100 grams of sugar contain 400 calories, but 100 grams of fat contains a whopping 900 calories.

Obesity occurs due to fat accumulation subcutaneously and even in and around the visceral organs. However, burning these stored calories is challenging and requires much effort.

Thus, if you start with thirty minutes of exercise and you are obese, you might not notice much weight loss even after twelve weeks.

However, that does not mean nothing has changed. Remember that you will not see how the fat accumulated in your liver and around various internal organs is reduced and how these fat stores shrink. Thus, just keep exercising, and you will start seeing visible changes in the body.

How fast you see results often depends on how obese you were when starting to exercise. Most people begin experiencing change after two to three weeks of moderate-intensity training.

Certainly, when aiming for weight loss, it's important to bear in mind that by burning just seven hundred extra calories per week, you could potentially shed approximately ten pounds over the course of a year. That said, it's understandable that most individuals aspire to achieve more significant weight loss results. This suggests that setting more ambitious targets becomes essential.

We recommend being patient. If you make weight loss plans that are too grandiose, you are likely to not achieve them and thus become discouraged and leave physical training. Instead, focus on regular physical training and slowly increase the length and intensity of the training period over the months. Results will definitely follow.

Everyone who has exercised regularly for months has experienced benefits or weight loss. Some people just need more time to make lifestyle changes. For example, it takes time to reduce daily calorie intake, stop binge eating, reduce the habit of munching most of the time, and train five times or more a week.

Every drop of sweat you shed will ultimately bring you closer to your goal.

Keep in mind that with every pound of weight loss, you are significantly reducing your risk of metabolic disorders, diabetes, heart problems, joint disorders, dementia, and even cancer.

Suppose you are looking to lose weight fast—in three months, let's say. Yes, that is also possible, and it is not as challenging as it may sound. For quick weight loss, one might consider significantly cutting down total calorie intake for twelve weeks, perhaps switching to an 800-calorie diet for twelve weeks, but no longer than that, as it may be harmful to health. Start exercising for thirty minutes a day and progress to sixty minutes daily at the same time, and results are almost guaranteed.

However, once you have made some progress, you can become less strict with yourself and switch to a diet that is moderately rich in calories, consuming perhaps 1,200 to 1,400 calories a day. At the same time, continue to train for sixty minutes five times a week. Ensure that your training is the right mix of aerobic/cardio and resistance training.

When it comes to exercise, it just takes time to get used to it. Thus, if you stick to your exercise program, you might make more meaningful progress after a few months. After a few months, you will have the ability to train for longer hours. Moreover, you will have more voluminous muscles that can burn a greater number of calories in less time. Exercise increases your mileage and boosts your engine's capacity or horsepower. Thus, as you progress, you can burn calories more quickly.

Of course, there will be periods when you will feel as if you are not making any progress. Remember that such phases come and go. All you need to do is stick to your training. If required, you might make some changes, like engaging in different exercises and changing exercise intensity.

Finally, remember that weight loss is one thing, and maintaining body weight after shedding several pounds is even more challenging.

Hence, we repeatedly mention treating exercise as akin to food and sleep, something that is part of your daily regime.

Of course, there will be days when you may not feel like training, and taking breaks now and then is OK. Do not do so for prolonged intervals, however, as returning to exercise may then become very difficult.

Quite commonly, people take a break from exercise and then fail to return, thus losing all the hard-gained results.

So exercise daily, be disciplined, see how your body transforms for the better, enjoy your new shape, and stay motivated.

All people are born equal, but how they look later in life depends on how much they sweat. Weight loss is even more important for older adults, who are more likely to develop chronic ailments.

Reduces Risk of Chronic Health Conditions and Diseases

A sedentary lifestyle is increasingly recognized as a significant health risk, comparable to the dangers of smoking. It's crucial to understand the importance of regular physical activity in mitigating these risks and promoting overall health.

If you do not move sufficiently, it increases the risk of almost every health disorder. It can even suppress immunity and make you more vulnerable to infectious diseases.

Exercise is especially good at lowering the risk of noninfectious or noncommunicable disorders. Since noncommunicable disorders are the major cause of mortality, exercise can be seen as the most effective preventive measure and remedy. No known pill or supplement can help like exercise.

Regretfully, most people do not start exercising, as taking pills a few times a day or using supplements is easier. And yet, without exercise, these measures have limited benefits.

Exercise is especially good for your heart and blood vessels. One-third of the adults live with high blood pressure and high cholesterol, and they ultimately develop heart diseases prematurely.

Exercise can make your heart stronger, increase vascular elasticity, normalize lipid metabolism, and thus help prevent hypertension, dyslipidemia, and coronary vascular disease.

Even those already living with these conditions can benefit from exercise. High blood pressure or cholesterol is not a reason to not engage in physical activity. In fact, many may be able to correct these health issues solely through dietary measures and exercise. Let food and exercise be thy medicine.

Heart disease is also not a contraindication for exercise, though it means that one should start any exercise program under medical supervision.

People should further understand that some of the most dreaded noninfectious diseases, such as stroke, are also a kind of cardiovascular ailment. Thus, if you train daily, you are not just minimizing your risk of a heart attack but also significantly reducing your risk of stroke.

Another big problem in modern society is the increasing prevalence of diabetes. Ten to twelve percent of the population is already living with diabetes. However, this is not a complete picture. Another 30 percent of the population is living with borderline diabetes or prediabetes. These are massive numbers.[22]

That means that 40 percent of the population has an abnormal metabolism. Fortunately, 80 percent of these people can reverse their condition merely through exercise and a balanced diet.

Almost every nation in the world has carried out many diabetes prevention studies. Nearly all studies, whether done in Finland, the

US, or India, have similar findings: exercise can cut down the risk of developing diabetes in most people. Not only that, but exercise is also a more effective way to reverse prediabetes than medications.

It is regretful that most people view exercise as something challenging. Furthermore, they believe that exercise only helps after a long time or they would only benefit by engaging in an extensive exercise program. These are false perceptions.

Exercise starts helping and reducing the risk of diseases from day one, though you might not feel it. If you experience reduced body weight, blood pressure, and blood glucose after a few months, it is a result of that first step. The benefits of exercise accumulate over time, quite like fats accumulate gradually.

Merely staying active for thirty minutes a day, like engaging in brisk walking, is enough to reduce your risk of various health conditions significantly. However, sixty minutes a day is even better.

Similarly, reducing body weight by 5 to 7 percent may cut down your risk of heart attack and diabetes by half. Of course, this is the case if the weight loss is due to exercise.[23] [24]

Exercise can help in the most unexpected ways. Some health benefits may be experienced much later in life. After all, the young body, heart, liver, bones, and joints work wonderfully even under much stress. Yet as you start getting older, you need more maintenance.

Those who do not exercise in adulthood are more likely to develop osteoarthritis later in life. In addition, they are more likely to have weak bones, osteoporosis, hormonal issues, and other problems.

Exercise also ensures that your liver remains in peak health. In addition, it can minimize the risk of nonalcoholic fatty liver disease, the leading cause of sluggish liver and the most prominent risk factor for liver cancer.

Exercise further ensures gut motility and bile juices, and other digestive enzymes keep flowing as usual, even as you age. That is why we said that exercise is not just about weight loss or building muscles; most of its health benefits remain invisible, but they are ultimately felt.

Physical activity is one of the most effective ways to reduce your cancer risk.

Exercise results in numerous changes in the body, including hormonal, immunological, and metabolic changes. Researchers have found that exercise can significantly reduce the risk of some of the most common types of cancers, like breast, lung, bladder, colon, endometrium, esophagus, kidney, and stomach cancer.

Though there are many reasons why cancer incidence is rising globally, the lack of physical activity is one of the significant contributing factors.

So, yes, exercise is the best health insurance. It ensures that you do not fall ill, unlike insurance bought through monetary means, which helps you get medical help but cannot prevent all the pain of being ill.

Improves Mood

Have you ever thought that your habit of procrastination and constantly worrying about various small matters may be the result of a lack of sufficient physical activity? Yes, if you do not exercise, you are more likely to check multiple times if you have closed your door. You are more likely to spend time worrying about various minor problems. According to a study by Sharma, Madaan, and Petty, regular physical activity can significantly mitigate these behaviors by reducing stress and enhancing mood.

Anxiety is the most common mental health issue. Those who do not exercise are more likely to live with more severe forms of anxiety. Of course, worrying about various matters is fine and normal.

However, worrying so much that it starts interfering with your life is not normal.

Anxiety is not a fear of real threats but rather a fear of perceived threats. If you keep track of things, you have no doubt noticed that most of your worries are futile. All those negative thoughts are just unnecessary fears. In reality, things usually turn out to be much better.

Want to stop worrying? Those sedative pills that keep your nerves calm are not the answer. Instead, those pills, or even supplements, may close one hole in the boat by creating yet another. Relying on such substances for managing fears can harm your health in various ways. Although they are not going to improve your mood, they might provide temporary relief.

Using substances, medications, and supplements to tackle anxiety is just like riding the waves. Unfortunately, these waves keep returning, becoming more prominent each day.

So be strong, act, start exercising, and experience the magic. How quickly you benefit depends on how long you have lived with the condition. Your mood will improve from the first workout session. However, overcoming severe anxiety may require a few months of dedication. [25]

Another mood issue, a little less common than anxiety but more severe, is depression. It is a condition that causes people to just stop enjoying life and look at everything in a pessimistic way. Those who suffer from depression lose interest in every activity and even in life. As a result, many may develop suicidal thoughts, and some may listen to those ugly thoughts.

Depression is a complex and multifaceted condition that can affect anyone, regardless of their physical health, wealth, or success. It's a common misconception that this condition only impacts those who are visibly struggling; in reality, it can also affect individuals who appear outwardly happy and successful. The tragic loss of Robin Williams, a beloved comedian known for his vibrant persona, highlights the profound and often hidden impact of mental health issues.

While Robin Williams was celebrated for his incredible talent, his struggles with mental health were less visible. It's crucial to recognize that mental well-being is as important as physical health. Regular exercise is one of many tools that can contribute positively to mental health management. However, it's important to remember that mental health conditions require a comprehensive approach, often including medical care, therapy, support networks, and lifestyle changes.

Yes, exercise helps you significantly reduce the risk of major depression. Even if you develop depression, it will be much milder. Exercise means more endorphins, dopamine, serotonin, and oxytocin, resulting in greater pleasure from simple things in life.

There are many possible reasons for falling into depression. Often, people have real reasons—threats, troubles, losses, grief, and so on. However, the development of these mental health disorders still has much to do with how you tackle those problems. Exercise provides you with that much-needed energy to keep going, forget pains, and restart enjoying your life.

Of course, even a drink will help you overcome anxiety or depression. However, your troubles will return the next day. With such measures, you may become bipolar, a person who is excited one day and depressed another.

If you want to achieve that internal calmness and satisfaction from life, move frequently and extensively, make your body sweat and your heart pump a lot of blood to your brain, and then see the magic happen.

Certain traumatic experiences can lead to nightmares, fears, and anxiety, a condition known as PTSD (posttraumatic stress disorder) in medical terms. By redirecting your energy toward activities such as weight lifting or running, you are more likely to experience a sense of calmness and enjoy improved sleep.

If you go to doctors, they treat those conditions. They prescribe antianxiety drugs, medications that help overcome depression. However, these medications have numerous side effects. They never treat the root cause of your mood disorders. All they do is temporarily alter your brain's functioning at the expense of your long-term health.

Most studies show that these medications are only good for some severe cases. In addition, most people would benefit more from changing their thoughts than resorting to drugs.

Exercise helps you start thinking differently and viewing the world in a better light. Start exercising to enjoy life's simple pleasures each day, the things we might not notice when living with toxic thought patterns.

In the olden days, people worked physically and did not know much about anxiety or depression. They never had time to worry so much or feel depressed. These were regarded as rare diseases in those good old days. After a hard working day, they ate and slept tight.

Those who do not move their muscles much during the day are not likely to have a good appetite for food or sleep. Exercise is the best appetizer in the world, and it renews your senses. It normalizes your appetite.

If you exercise, you are more likely to seek healthy foods; you are less likely to suffer from eating disorders, sleep issues, and problems.

Engaging in physical work or exercise can profoundly transform your experience of everyday meals. The satisfaction derived from eating after a day of physical activity is markedly different from that experienced amid a sedentary lifestyle. In contrast, those with less active lifestyles may often find themselves seeking pleasure in less healthy options like sodas, sweets, and foods high in salt and fat.

The impact of mental health conditions, including eating disorders and sleep disturbances, on overall health is frequently underestimated. Yet these issues play a crucial role in our well-being. Regular exercise stands out as a highly effective method for enhancing mental health.

Boosts Energy Levels

Lack of energy is one of the most common complaints these days. It is one of the reasons why many do not exercise without realizing that they will remain stuck in a vicious cycle if they do not start moving. No exercise means low energy, and low energy means no wish to exercise.

However, regretfully, people seek remedies for their low energy levels in the wrong things. They may visit doctors, talk to friends for health advice, and buy a heap of supplements. Those who have done these things know that they rarely help. Of course, it would help if the low energy level was due to some physical ailment or nutritional deficiencies. However, a low energy level is rarely due to some disorder. Instead, it is rather a kind of warning that if you do not start moving, your body will give up and develop some ailment.

Often, when people visit the doctor, they are prescribed dozens of lab tests, only to discover there's nothing wrong. Then doctors might prescribe supplements; even worse, they might prescribe antidepressants and similar drugs that only further complicate things.

If you seldom engage in physically demanding tasks, your body stops accumulating energy in your skeletal muscles. Instead, it stores most energy, such as fats, under your skin. You have to change all this and send the right signals to your body by exercising.

Of course, if most of your lab tests are normal, it does not indicate that all is well. Instead, it simply means that many health issues are still challenging to diagnose due to the lack of reliable biomarkers.

Many living with low energy are individuals suffering from chronic stress and low levels of inflammation. This means that the levels of various hormones are disrupted. Science has only started to realize that this prolonged low level of stress and inflammation is the main cause of many severe physical ailments.

So, listen to your body. If you lack energy, it is a signal to start exercising. Increased rest is not going to help in such instances.

For example, constant worries and stress may elevate cortisol levels. Cortisol increases blood glucose levels and may even increase energy levels a bit. However, if it remains constantly high, it depletes the body of vital energy sources.

So, instead of lying on the couch, watching television, or browsing the internet, get up, start moving, or even better, start jogging or running. Aerobic exercise is an excellent way to boost your energy levels.

If you find exercising boring, find some more exciting activity like cycling or swimming or playing sports. It is not important what activity you do but rather that you get started and experience a rush of energy over the course of a few days.

Of course, in many cases, doctors might have identified the cause of low energy. They might have told you that you have fibromyalgia or chronic fatigue syndrome. Even if you have these disorders, exercise is the best-known cure.

These conditions occur due to specific changes in the brain. Unfortunately, there is no drug therapy that can effectively cure them, nor any supplement that works in all cases.

In most cases, medications and supplements may help a bit. However, if you want to regain control of your life, start living without pain, and be full of energy, exercise is an effective remedy.

Promotes Better Sleep

Work out hard and sleep harder. Sleep is essential to staying healthy and resetting the brain and body. It is the time when regenerative processes occur at the fastest pace. That is why if you feel ill, just a bit of sleep often suffices to ensure that you start feeling better. There is definitely something magical about sleep.

Exercise will help you to fall asleep faster. Not only that, but it will also enhance sleep quality, which is equally essential. It is not sufficient to sleep seven hours a day; you must also sleep *well*.

During sleep, people go through multiple phases like light sleep, deep sleep, and REM (rapid eye movement) sleep, and these cycles repeat multiple times during the night. Each cycle has its role in human health.

REM may help the brain reorganize thoughts and information and allow you to mentally prepare for the next day. NREM (nonrapid eye movement) sleep is when most of the healing occurs. Regenerative processes occur quickly during deep sleep, though deep sleep only constitutes about 25 percent of the total sleep time.

If you work out, you will notice that you start sleeping better. These days, most people have wearables that can monitor sleep and give an idea of how you slept. If you do not have a wearable, invest in one, as it helps track workouts and activity levels during the day, as well as, more importantly, sleep.

Start exercising, and notice how your sleep scores improve over time.

Here, it is vital to understand that exercise may negatively impact your sleep due to body aches and fatigue in the early few weeks. That said, your sleep will considerably improve once you get used to a certain activity level.

Many adults have forgotten when they last had a sound and continuous sleep for several hours. Because many people find it hard to sleep and have too many worries, thoughts, and stresses, they frequently wake up during the night and have many other sleep issues. But, most people experience a significant change in sleep quality after starting to exercise.

There is a reason why we are focusing so much on the relationship between exercise and sleep. Sleep remains one of the neglected aspects of health. Indeed, poor sleep is not just suggestive of poor health; a lack of good night's sleep is also a risk factor for many health disorders.

A few years back, doctors considered sleep to be just one of the minor contributing factors to ill health. However, now studies show that poor sleep is one of the most significant factors behind different health disorders.

It is an independent risk factor for many disease conditions. This means that even if you improve different aspects of your life, take dietary measures, take health supplements, and so on, if you are not sleeping well, you are still at significant risk of metabolic disorders, mental health issues, and neurological conditions.

Now, doctors realize that sleep has a two-sided relationship with conditions like anxiety, depression, diabetes, and even auto-immune disorders. Poor health and the presence of any of these conditions result in poor sleep due to pain and other health issues. On the other hand, poor sleep also significantly increases the risk of these disorders.

To break this vicious cycle, a key strategy is to focus on enhancing the quality of your sleep.

While there are numerous approaches to improving sleep, one essential method you should not overlook is regular exercise. Incorporating physical activity into your routine can significantly contribute to better sleep quality.

Brings Back the Spark to Your Sex Life

There is a book called *The Hardness Factor: How to Achieve Your Best Health and Sexual Fitness at Any Age*. This book promoted one very good idea: that the penis is the barometer of a man's health.

The harder the man's erection, the healthier he is. And this is true to an extent.

Of course, this book is about males. When it comes to females, however, it would be correct to say that sexual desire may indicate the level of health.

Naturally, things are a little bit more complex with females due to menopause-related issues. Nonetheless, women benefit equally from exercise. For them, it leads to avoiding early menopause and the ability to enjoy sex after menopause.

I hope you get the point. For both men and women, their sex life, at least to a degree, indicates how well they are. Those who feel unwell not only experience poor sexual function but also have low sexual desire.

Exercise can improve both sexual desire and function. So before we discuss these topics further, it is vital to understand the difference.

Sexual desire, or libido, refers to the wish to have sex more frequently or regularly. Sexual function refers to the ability to have sex. Some may have a desire but struggle to have satisfactory sex. For example, men may struggle due to poor erection quality, and women due to vaginal dryness or other issues.

Libido, or sexual desire, is mainly the function of sex hormones. Thus, in men, it is primarily influenced by testosterone, and in women, by estrogen, progesterone, and testosterone. Things are more complex for women; they have testosterone in small amounts.

Exercise is one of the good ways to boost testosterone production, but it may also help maintain the level of various other hormones in females as well. Thus, it is the safest and most effective way to maintain hormonal health.

Still, there are other mechanisms also involved in sexual desire, like the autonomous nervous system and different neurotransmitters. Exercise ensures that these neurotransmitters are produced in optimal quantity, thus ensuring sexual desire and arousal.

Further, remember that exercise also considerably improves blood flow to the genitals, which may also influence the quality of sexual arousal. Additionally, exercise ensures that the body can sustain many enzymes that enhance blood flow to the genitals for longer, thus boosting both libido and sexual function.

Regretfully, the impact of exercise on men is a more-often-discussed topic. But exercise is equally good for both genders. One of the reasons men get greater attention is that sexual dysfunction in men is relatively visible. Men cannot pretend to have a hard erection.

If they do not get a hard erection, there is no way they can satisfy their partner. However, this does not mean that sexual dysfunction is not present in females.

Females struggle with sexual dysfunction equally, if not more. In addition, as they age, they have issues related to low hormones. This affects their genitals, increasing the risk of various problems, from vaginal dryness and poor blood flow to infections. Hence, females who exercise regularly are more likely to enjoy sex and have better sexual function.[26]

There is no doubt that, in the long run, exercise can have a massively positive impact on your sex life. Take the example of people living with obesity, diabetes, and cardiovascular issues. Sexual dysfunction is among the most significant problems among these people. Unfortunately, most men and women living with these health issues have a poor sex life. For many, a sex life is almost absent.

Exercise not only improves your sex hormone levels but also boosts the production of growth hormones, various other hormones, and enzymes.

This also means lower insulin resistance, higher metabolic rate, better musculoskeletal health, and higher endurance due to improved cardiovascular health.

People who exercise regularly react very differently to sexual arousal. They have a stronger desire and, more importantly, quick and more intense arousal. As a result, they can have sex for longer, resulting in greater satisfaction from the sexual act.

When it comes to the choice of exercise in this regard, we would like to emphasize that though exercises like Kegels are good, they will not help you if you have a poor fitness level. They are thus of secondary importance.

If you want to get fit, you should start with aerobic, HIIT, and resistance training to ensure complete fitness. Exercises like Kegels can only help those who are relatively fit.

For those living with sexual dysfunction or older adults, it is better to have a training program covering every fitness aspect. It is about building stamina, flexibility, and balance; improving cardiorespiratory health, joint health, mental focus, and more. Of course, focusing on core muscles may have some additional benefits in improving sexual performance.

Keep in mind that your sexual health is the barometer of your health. It is not just about hormones. That is why drugs like Viagra work. Such drugs do not contain any hormones; instead, they work on blood vessels. This is further proof that sexual function can only be improved through complete fitness.

Many people fail to improve their sex lives as they blame a lack of hormones. Of course, hormones have much to do with your sex life, but they are just one of the elements. If you have a perfectly good sex hormone level, this does not mean that you will automatically start enjoying sex or have sexual stamina.

Moreover, it is no secret that sex is also physically demanding. If you cannot run a couple of miles, do not expect to last long in bed. You will simply get tired, your heart will fail to manage the stress, your muscles will give up, and your blood vessels will not cope.

And, finally, remember that exercise will also improve your mood. You will have lower stress levels and can keep hormones like cortisol at low levels. Exercise is better for uplifting mood than cherries or strawberries.

Stress hormones are the biggest spoilers of sex life. Thus, exercise is not just about boosting different body functions. It is also about suppressing specific harmful bodily responses to ensure harmony and balance.

It's Fun and Helps One Socialize

It is not enough to be healthy or disease-free; having fun is also essential to staying happy. Exercise is a medium, but the ultimate reason to do physical activities is to be healthy, happy, and satisfied with life.

Further, we are social animals. Prolonged isolation is not good for our physical and mental well-being. And exercise can also help you socialize better.

Exercise is never intended to be boring, even if you are doing it alone. If it is dull and boring, you are doing it in the wrong way, and chances are that you won't be able to carry on for long. If you find exercising stressful and tedious, you must reconsider many factors.

Every person is different. Thus, there is no correct answer to the question of which exercise is the most fun. Some introverts may find greater enjoyment in jogging, listening to music, and spending time with themselves. For others, aerobic classes may provide greater satisfaction.

That is why mixing different exercises, like resistance training with aerobics or even sports training, is good. For example, you might train in a gym for five days a week and play tennis on weekends.

Whether you are an introvert or an extrovert, we highly recommend placing special emphasis on socialization. Ultimately, it holds significance. The people around you can offer assistance, guidance, and more. Even engaging in simple conversations and sharing your feelings with others can be beneficial.

Of course, when we say that exercise is fun and helps us socialize, that does not mean that socialization happens solely while exercising.

For example, you might prepare for 10K and then make it a habit to participate in various running events organized throughout the country. This would allow you to travel, discover new places, and make new friends.

If you exercise and stay fit, you can join hiking clubs and go for long walks on weekends or whenever you have time.

Here, we are suggesting that you stop viewing exercise as something boring. Lifting weights alone or running on a treadmill are not the only ways to exercise. Likewise, working out all the time alone is not a good idea.

When exercising, think of both your physical and mental health. For example, you might join yoga classes and make friends there with similar hobbies. Moreover, those engaged in sports are more likely to have a healthy lifestyle.

The options are endless, so just use your imagination. Always try to engage in different kinds of physical activities. Do not neglect the fun side of sports and exercise.

Exercise is not just about building physical abilities or your body shape. It must include activities that ensure mental well-being. Moreover, people are increasingly feeling lonely these days due to the ever-increasing use of gadgets, work-from-home practices, and other reasons.

So next time you go to the gym, smile, try to socialize, and say hello to others. If you do not have a training buddy, finding one is not that difficult. There are many people looking for training buddies, and you just need to break the ice and take the initiative.

Exercise Is the Best Antiaging Medicine

Aging is unpreventable, but it can be slowed down. Exercise is one of the most reliable ways to age gracefully. Unfortunately, some middle-aged people have ailing hearts and joints and other issues. And then there are those who live as if they are twenty years old. In most cases, significant differences between two adults are the result of one exercising and the other not.

Of course, many factors decide how you age, including diet and genetics. Nonetheless, physical activity, or lack of it, is the single most important deciding factor.

Someone rightly said that as we start to grow older, we begin losing the ability to do things we do not regularly do. Thus, if you do not run or jump as you age, you won't be able to do that again.

Without exercise, you will lose many skills and physical abilities forever. After that, there is no going back. We are not saying this to frighten you; it is a harsh reality.

That is why exercise plans for older adults must differ from those for young adults. In the case of older adults, an exercise plan must contain different kinds of physical activities. One must avoid overinvesting in a single type of activity.

Let's take the example of CrossFit training, which is quite good for older adults. If you want to age slowly and gracefully, you need to do all sorts of different physical activities and movements. You need to keep both your muscles and your joints strong, maintain balance and flexibility, and boost your mental alertness.

Of course, aging is not just about physical fitness; it is about many other things, like skin elasticity, memory, energy level, being free of disease, and more. It is also about staying strong for longer and having higher endurance levels.

So, yes, exercise is the only known elixir. Regretfully, the chances are close to nil that scientists will ever discuss any magic potion providing immortality and youth forever. Instead, try to do what is known to considerably increase lifespan, youth, and vitality—that is, start investing your time in exercise.

The National Institute on Aging recommends that all adults engage in four types of exercises: *endurance, balance, strength, and flexibility training.*[27]

The message is pretty simple. There is no secret to prolonging youth. So just find the right kind of exercise, one you think you can do daily.

As we have seen, exercise is the most effective way to boost the flow of different hormones, including sex hormones. It also helps keep neurotransmitter production in your brain, ensuring sound mental health.

Exercise Helps Prevent Cognitive Decline

Physical agility is good, but the brain is the main thing. The brain makes you what and who you are. That is why there is an old saying that "if money is lost, nothing is lost; if health is lost, something is lost; if character is lost, everything is lost."

People have a habit of viewing exercise as something for physical well-being, and they completely forget about the benefits of exercise for brain health.

However, this discussion is now more relevant than ever before. As humans have started to live longer, declining cognition has become a major issue.

Just consider conditions like Alzheimer's and other forms of dementia. Dementia is now among the leading causes of disability and even death in developed nations. However, more than a hundred years of research have failed to find the real cause of increased dementia risk.

It is pretty likely that we might be overlooking a factor that may be contributing significantly to dementia, which is a lack of physical activity.[28]

It is interesting to note that dementia is rarely diagnosed in those under fifty. However, now researchers know that it starts much earlier. Indeed, dementia perhaps begins a decade or two before its diagnosis.

This means that some of the early changes characteristic of dementia start occurring in the brain in your thirties. This is the age when many people stop being active and start abusing substances and even food.

This explains why exercise should be a lifelong habit. Do not wait for something to go wrong, and then start exercising. Remember that reversing all the ill effects of years of neglect is not possible in many instances—always remember the legacy effect.

If you exercise daily at a young age, there is less chance you will develop dementia.

Of course, focusing too much on dementia alone would be unwise. A significant issue in older adults is age-related cognitive decline. It affects almost everyone as they age. However, the severity of the condition depends on how active your lifestyle is.

Do not forget to exercise when young to prevent forgetfulness when old and frail.

Those who stay active at a young age and keep training as they grow older are less likely to have any significant cognitive decline.

For scientific-minded people, it is worth knowing that regular exercise prevents the shrinking of the hippocampus, along with other brain areas participating in critical body functions, to a significant degree.

Exercise helps preserve gray matter and prevents the degradation of white matter in the brain.

Regular physical activity improves blood flow and energy production in the brain. This stimulates various brain areas. Thus, if you stay inactive, many brain areas start degrading fast. Exercise sends signals to the brain that various brain centers are still needed. That is why physical training has such a rejuvenating effect. But of course, to stay young for longer, you must send these signals to various parts of the brain more frequently.

Exercise helps maintain brain abilities in other ways, too. For example, physically active individuals remain socially active, communicate more with others, have better emotional health, and are more likely to engage in tasks demanding higher brain centers. So exercise keeps the brain trained directly and indirectly.

Remember the age-old saying, "A healthy brain resides in a healthy body." Our ancestors noticed the relationship between a healthy body and a healthy mind long ago. These are centuries-old observations that do not necessarily need any scientific proof. They have been proven over time.

To stay mentally alert and young, start moving, engage in physical activity, and have fun.

Good for Bone Health

Almost everyone knows that exercise builds lean mass or muscles. However, most people do not realize that exercise also builds or strengthens bones, promoting their remodeling and causing massive changes.

Just consider weight lifters. Their bones would crack due to mechanical stress if they grew only muscles. However, this does not happen as bones grow along with muscles, tendons, and ligaments. This means that resistance training helps build bones.

Despite what most people think, bones are not inert. On the contrary, they change all the time and are metabolically very dynamic structures. Two kinds of cells, osteoclasts and osteoblasts, ensure bone health.

Osteoclasts remove old and damaged bone parts and cells, whereas osteoclasts continually keep adding new mass to the bones.

Together, these cells ensure that bones keep evolving according to their needs.

This means that people can build not only muscles but also bones. In addition, all exercise forms have an impact on bone health. Thus, exercise can increase bone mineralization, strengthen bone, reduce fracture risk, and help prevent conditions like osteoarthritis.

Put another way, exercise can help treat osteoarthritis, as joint disorders are not a contraindication for exercise. If you have swollen joints, you only need to be careful and avoid high-impact activities like jumping. That said, most people do not realize that exercise is the most effective way to manage joint disorders.[29]

Most guidelines say that exercise should be part of joint disorder treatments, whether joint pain is due to osteoarthritis, rheumatoid arthritis, or other factors.

If you exercise, your body secretes more osteocalcin, ensuring more significant bone mineralization. However, that is not all, as this hormone has many other health benefits. Osteocalcin can lower blood sugar levels, help prevent diabetes, and promote fat burning, thus helping overcome obesity. Not only that, but osteocalcin also appears to interact with sex hormones; it may even boost their production.

It is essential to understand that your bones secrete hormones or hormonelike substances that have many health effects. Osteocalcin is just one of the examples of hormones with widespread health effects. However, there are many other hormones secreted by bones. Therefore, remember that bones also have an endocrinal function, and exercise helps normalize it.

But wait, that is not all. The truth is that bones play a more significant role in health and well-being than skeletal muscles. We must not forget that it is the bones, or bone marrow—a kind of soft tissue inside the bones—that produces red and white blood cells.

So, good bone health means that you are less likely to have blood-related issues and more likely to have good immunity. After all, every immune cell is generated by bone and then might mature in other body tissues.

You are entirely wrong if you still view bones as inert structures that merely support your body and provide a shape. Bones are also rich in stem cells. These unique cells can be converted into any other kind of body cell. Hence, bones play an important role in regenerative processes in the body.

Finally, do not forget that bones store vital nutrients. They store ions like calcium, magnesium, phosphorus, and other minerals. They release these minerals when and as needed.

Every time you run or pick up weights, remember that you are not only building muscles or burning fats but also stimulating bone remodeling.

In fact, bone remodeling due to regular exercise may have the greatest impact on health and well-being. And yet, bone health remains a neglected topic as changes in the bone are not visible to the naked eye like changes in muscle or fat mass.

You are as old as your bones. Bones are a direct reflection of your true metabolic age.

So next time you run, pick up weights, kick a soccer ball, or dance, keep in mind that you are not just making your heart pump and muscles work; you are doing good for your bones too.

Helps Reverse or Treat Disease Conditions

It is never too late to get started with exercise, even if you are living with some severe ailment.

One of the problems is that doctors and health experts continue to emphasize that exercise can help prevent disorders (which is definitely true). However, they are not telling people that exercise can also be medicine and can help treat or reverse ailments, often causing prolonged disease remission.

This is essential to understand that many people start exercising quite late when they are diagnosed with some severe ailment. But exercise is beneficial even if you have been diagnosed with a nonsevere disease condition, and it can help treat or reverse most disease conditions.

Of course, if you are diagnosed with a disease condition, you may need some medical advice before starting the exercise program. This does not mean it is something to be neglected. Exercise can be beneficial even if you are living with something as severe as cancer or a cardiovascular disorder.

However, exercise is relatively more beneficial in treating specific ailments. For example, it is especially good for managing chronic metabolic disorders.

Just take the example of diabetes. Doctors may fail to tell you that most guidelines, like those of the American Diabetes

Association (ADA), clearly say that prediabetes and mild diabetes must be managed initially through lifestyle interventions like dietary measures and exercise and that using medications in the early stages is not essential.

Moreover, new studies show that if you exercise, you will not only lower your blood glucose but can also achieve prolonged diabetes remission. If you start the right kind of exercise program early enough, before irreversible changes have occurred in your body, you can nearly cure your diabetes through exercise.

Guidelines for hypertension are similar. The American Heart Association (AHA) clearly says that mild hypertension should be managed through exercise. In addition, it clearly states that it is possible to manage the condition during the early stages without medications.

The AHA came up with the recommendation that all adults must engage in at least thirty minutes of moderate-intensity exercise daily.[11]

It is regretful that very few people prefer giving lifestyle interventions a try. However, as we have already stated, most people find it relatively simple to take a pill daily and can even shift the responsibility for their health to the health care provider in this way.

Meanwhile, the chronic care model clearly says that in chronic ailments, the patient is primarily responsible for managing the condition, and doctors can only assist them in achieving their health targets.

The problem with all this research regarding the management of these chronic conditions is that it remains inaccessible to most people. Doctors have done the studies, and they know the realities. However, they lack time to explain these findings to their patients. They are too busy to create and monitor dietary and exercise programs.

There are other specialists that can help, like diabetes educators. But unfortunately, they, too, have not been able to fulfill their roles fully.

The truth is that education in managing chronic ailments through exercise and diet is essential for all chronic diseases.

Take the example of depression. We already mentioned that exercise is good for mental health and can help prevent anxiety and depression.

However, what if a person is already living with depression? Exercise can be the single most effective remedy. Yes, exercise can help one overcome depression entirely and forever.

Again, discussing a medical approach to treating depression is not the subject of this book. Nevertheless, it is vital that our readers know that medical research suggests that all those antidepressants (medical drugs) do not appear to help with mild to moderate depression. Instead, they are mainly effective in a small number of people living with severe depression.

The best treatment for mild to moderate depression is to change your thought patterns. Doctors help achieve this with cognitive behavior therapy. Regular exercise is another effective way to overcome depression. It can help manage the root cause of the condition as it can boost the production of neurotransmitters, help overcome neuroinflammation, and help alter thought patterns.

The truth is that exercise must be a part of the treatment of most noncommunicable diseases. It is also suitable for cardiovascular ailments (of course, always start training under medical supervision), joint issues, addiction treatment, dementia, Parkinson's, and much more.

One final piece of advice: remember that although exercise is quite good for chronic noninfectious diseases, it also has a role in lowering the risk of mortality due to infections. Those who exercise regularly are less likely to develop severe flu, COVID-19, and other respiratory infections. And they are less likely to be hospitalized or die due to these infections.

Increases Self-Esteem and Helps One Look Good

We have mentioned multiple times in this book that the most important reason for exercising is to improve health, especially metabolic health. Such improvements may not be visible to the naked eye immediately, but they occur from day one. Even a single exercise session is a step in the right direction.

However, we cannot neglect that one of the most popular reasons to get started with exercise is not health concerns but rather a wish to achieve an attractive body. This is not only the most popular reason for people to start exercising, but it is also highly motivating.

Many people are motivated to exercise by the desire to improve their physical appearance, including achieving a well-defined body and perhaps even six-pack abs. This aspiration is understandable as a more attractive appearance often correlates with increased sexual appeal, tapping into one of our most basic instincts.

While the quest for a better physique is a common reason to engage in physical activity, it's important to emphasize the myriad health benefits that exercise offers. This has been a focus throughout our discussion because understanding the health implications of exercise is crucial.

It's also essential to understand that though having a fit and toned body is often associated with good health, this isn't always the case. Take professional bodybuilders, for instance; despite their remarkable physiques, they may not necessarily epitomize overall health due to factors like overtraining and maintaining extremely low body fat percentages.

In your pursuit of an aesthetically pleasing body, remember that your overall health should always be the priority. Striving to enhance your sexual attractiveness is perfectly valid, but it should not come at the cost of your health. Therefore, avoid the temptation of shortcuts like banned substances. True fitness encompasses both external appearance and internal well-being.

Lowering body fats to extremely low levels is harmful. In other words, too much body fat is bad for health, but too little is also dangerous. For example, in females, most testosterone is produced in fat cells by converting estrogens. Thus, low fat mass results in low testosterone, poor bone health, and mental health issues.

It is a positive thing to look in the mirror more often, take images, and focus on improving your shape. However, at the same time, keep in mind that the primary target should be better health.

When you are in good shape, you are naturally more energized and mobile, and more importantly, you have higher self-esteem. In addition, you are more likely to make friends. Of course, all these things also translate into better health.

So our recommendation is simple: exercise regularly to improve health. If you work out regularly, it will naturally lead to a good body shape. However, avoid focusing too much on that as it may sometimes harm your health.

Avoid unhealthy methods of improving your shape like strict dieting, trying to get rid of the last drop of fat in your body, using drugs and medications, and other unhealthy means.

Instead, focus on being healthy yet attractive.

As we are here touching on the subject of the difference between being in good shape and being healthy, we would also like to remind you that many of the people seen in the posters and adverts might look amazing but are not essentially healthy.

In fact, most professional sportspeople are not healthy due to overtraining, which causes excessive stress on the body. They also go through many traumas in their life and have many other issues. For example, many of them have a so-called athletic heart. Others develop neurodegenerative diseases due to brain micro-trauma and have many other similar issues. The truth is that many of those famous people we see with impressive physical capabilities are not healthy and do not necessarily live long. Moreover, they often have to spend massive amounts on medical bills when they get old.

The Bottom Line on Exercise

Have we mentioned all the significant benefits associated with exercise? Definitely not. Exercise affects each of the body's cells. Its benefits go deep inside the skin and are much more profound than visible changes. So even if you do not lose a pound, you are still doing a great service to your body by exercising.

The whole purpose of telling you about the health benefits of exercise is to help you develop greater insight. You know that exercise is an essential element of modern human life as people do not need to move much to seek food and other resources. They thus need to compensate for that immobility by moving intentionally and by engaging in exercise.

You are not just burning fats or strengthening skeletal and cardiac muscles when you exercise. You are also changing how cells produce energy, how mitochondria work, how genes express themselves, and what proteins the endoplasmic reticulum produces.

Exercising forces every cell organelle and billions of genes inside your body to change their behavior. Even ions like calcium and sodium behave differently.

So, who said that you could not control the working of your cells or that genes cannot be modified? What if we told you that exercise could alter your genes and you could pass those healthy changes onto the next generation? What if we told you that by exercising, you are ensuring the good health of the next generation too? Of course, that is if you start exercising early enough.

If that all sounds like an exaggeration to you, then it is time for you to learn more about epigenetics—a science that shows that human behavior can alter gene expression. For example, you can silence specific genes and activate other genes merely through your lifestyle choices; these changes in gene expression can be passed down to the next generation.

This means that exercising can positively influence every body function, improve your survivability, reduce the risk of various health disorders, and allow you to become healthy. Moreover, exercise, if done regularly and habitually, has the power to change your genes and reprogram them. Therefore, it can make you healthy from the inside.

That is why you should never judge your efforts after a few weeks of workouts. Do not think your scale is telling you all the truth or that measurements like biceps circumference can help you understand the health benefits of exercise.

There is no way to measure millions of small changes that occur in the body every time you exercise. However, together, these changes can alter the course of your life. This can create a healthy you, a person resilient to diseases, infections, mental health issues, and more.

Once you recognize all the positive outcomes that come from exercising, you'll understand that saving on health insurance is just one of the many advantages. Nevertheless, the reduction in health insurance expenses is a valuable addition to the array of benefits that exercise provides.

That is why we say *exercise is the best health insurance.*

Even in the presence of exercise, we still need health insurance, however. So let's look further into the subject, see how it helps one stay healthy, consider its pros and cons, and explore how you can save on health insurance through exercise.

END-OF-MODULE-V ACTIVITIES

Discovering the Full Spectrum of Exercise Benefits

Personal Exploration: Reflect on your understanding of the various benefits of regular physical activity before and after this module. Identify which benefit(s) of exercise you find most motivating for your personal situation.

_____

_____

_____

_____

_____

_____

_____

_____

_____

_____

_____

Knowledge Application: Based on what you've learned, draft a plan to incorporate a balanced exercise routine into your life. Consider including elements that address weight control, chronic disease prevention, mental health, sleep improvement, and sexual health.

_____

_____

_____

_____

_____

_____

_____

_____

_____

_____

_____

_____

Action Plan: Implement your exercise plan for a week, focusing on how each activity contributes to the different benefits discussed in the module. Pay attention to changes in your physical health, mood, sleep quality, and overall energy levels.

_____

_____

_____

_____

_____

_____

_____

_____

_____

_____

_____

_____

_____

_____

Reflective Journaling: Keep a daily journal during the week, documenting your exercise activities and their immediate and perceived long-term benefits. Note any challenges you faced and how you addressed them.

_____

_____

_____

_____

_____

_____

_____

_____

_____

_____

_____

_____

_____

_____

Review and Adaptation: At the end of the week, review your experiences and journal entries. Assess the effectiveness of your plan in addressing the comprehensive benefits of exercise. Modify your plan for ongoing improvement and sustainability.

END-OF-MODULE QUIZ

1. **Question:** What is the primary benefit of regular physical activity for weight management?

   A) Increases appetite

   B) Helps in burning calories and boosts metabolism

   C) Decreases muscle mass

   D) No impact on weight

2. **Question:** How does regular exercise impact mental health?

   A) Increases stress levels

   B) Has no effect on mental health

   C) Reduces symptoms of anxiety and depression

   D) Only improves physical health

3. **Question:** What effect does physical activity have on sleep?

   A) Worsens sleep quality

   B) Shortens sleep duration

   C) Improves sleep quality

   D) No effect on sleep

4. **Question:** Regular exercise is beneficial for cardiovascular health because it:

   A) Weakens the heart muscle

   B) Reduces blood circulation

   C) Increases blood pressure

   D) Strengthens the heart and improves circulation

5. **Question:** How does regular exercise affect the aging process?

   A) Accelerates aging

   B) Has no impact on aging

   C) Slows down aging and reduces age-related diseases

   D) Only affects physical appearance

ANSWERS

1. B) Helps in burning calories and boosts metabolism
2. C) Reduces symptoms of anxiety and depression
3. C) Improves sleep quality
4. D) Strengthens the heart and improves circulation
5. C) Slows down aging and reduces age-related diseases

MODULE VI

HEALTH INSURANCE

The US is among the largest and most populated nations in the world. Thus, naturally, it is a nation of diversity. The same is true for its health care system and insurance system. Things are pretty complex and far from ideal.

This country holds the record for the highest per capita health care expenditure globally. On average, health care costs here are roughly twice those in EU nations, highlighting a substantial difference.

However, what is worrisome is that despite Americans spending so much on health care and insurance, they are not necessarily getting the best health care services. Life expectancy in the US is not higher than that in most European nations.

The US is also an innovative nation. It can provide the most advanced health care services, yet these services remain unreachable for many of its citizens.

It has some of the largest pharmaceutical companies in the world, and yet the average cost of medications here is among the highest in the world. The interference of Big Pharma in every aspect of health care is an entirely different subject, and much has been written about it.

Similarly, there are many insurance plans, some of which are brilliantly conceived. Yet things are a bit confusing, as many health insurance options exist. In addition, Public and private players play a significant role.

To add to the confusion, the US has publicly funded insurance coverage, private coverage, and more. There are many subtypes of insurance in each category. Despite the existence of so many different kinds of health insurance, more than half of the population is unsatisfied with their insurance plan as it does not provide sufficient coverage.

It is no surprise that things keep changing in the US. New legislation is introduced every few years, though it does not seem to solve this chronic problem. Hence, 14 to 15 percent of the US population remains uninsured.

Generally, private plans provide better coverage, and they are associated with better health outcomes. That is expected as private insurance plans have higher payouts to doctors compared to public coverage. But those private plans are quite expensive and even unaffordable for many.

Moreover, health experts think that these private insurance plans are fueling the rise in health care costs. It is no secret that health care costs in the US have risen disproportionately to income. This trend has continued since the 1970s. Thus, paying for a good private health care plan is a significant financial burden even for those with a six-figure income.

Understanding insurance plans in the US might be complex, but exercising is not. Thus, it is the best health insurance. In addition, exercising makes you considerably less likely to require one of these various health insurance plans.

Types of Health Insurance

Health insurance has a significant history, with the origins of early private insurance companies in the US dating back to the mid-nineteenth century. These early forms of insurance primarily focused on covering injuries and accidents rather than a comprehensive range of health services. It wasn't until the twentieth century that health insurance companies began offering plans covering a broader spectrum of health care services. The health insurance industry has evolved considerably over time, reflecting changes in health care needs and societal values.

Health care coverage plans broadly fall into two categories: *public health coverage* and *private health coverage.*

These plans differ in the way they are funded and managed. Both public and private health coverage have their advantages and disadvantages. Public plans are crucial for providing access to health care for those who might otherwise be unable to afford it, but they may have limitations in coverage and provider networks. Private plans offer more extensive coverage and flexibility but at a higher cost, which can be a barrier for many individuals. The choice between public and private health insurance often depends on an individual's health care needs, financial situation, and eligibility for public programs.

Public Health Care Coverage

Public health care coverage in the US encompasses various programs designed to cater to different segments of the population, particularly those considered vulnerable. These segments include older adults, children, veterans, and certain demographic groups that might have specific health care needs. Key public healthcare programs include Medicare, Medicaid, the Children's Health Insurance Program (CHIP), TRICARE, the Veterans Health Administration, and the Indian Health Service.

Medicare is a federal program primarily serving individuals aged sixty-five and older, but it also covers younger individuals with certain disabilities and diseases. Medicare provides coverage for people with end-stage renal disease (ESRD) and amyotrophic lateral sclerosis (ALS). It is known for significantly improving access to health care for its enrollees, including previously uninsured individuals.

Medicaid is a public assistance program, not a conventional insurance program. It provides comprehensive health coverage to eligible low-income adults, children, pregnant women, elderly adults, and people with disabilities. Funded jointly by the federal and state governments, Medicaid is administered at the state level with adherence to federal guidelines.

The program includes individuals with incomes up to 138 percent of the federal poverty level, a threshold that was expanded in many states under the Affordable Care Act (ACA). While Medicaid is income-based, it ensures consistent and essential health coverage for its enrollees. That said, the continuity of Medicaid coverage can be affected by changes in an individual's financial situation or alterations in state-level policies.

CHIP provides low-cost health coverage to children in families that earn too much to qualify for Medicaid but not enough to afford private coverage. It covers a broad range of services designed to meet children's unique health needs.

TRICARE provides health benefits for US Armed Forces military personnel, retirees, and their dependents.

The Veterans Health Administration offers a comprehensive health care system for eligible military veterans at VA medical centers and outpatient clinics.

Indian Health Service provides healthcare services to eligible American Indians and Alaska Natives.

Each of these public health coverage programs has specific eligibility criteria and benefits, aiming to ensure that different population groups receive the necessary health care services.

Private Health Coverage

As we can see, public health care is affordable, but it is only for the most vulnerable population groups. The majority of the US population does not fall into those categories. Thus, for most people, private health insurance is the way forward. It provides good health care coverage, but, again, good plans cost a lot.

There are nearly one thousand health insurance companies in the US. However, a handful of them dominate the market, thus dictating its terms and controlling it. In addition, there is a kind of monopoly of a few private companies. These companies can influence health care in many ways, including raising costs.

Data show that around 60 percent of Americans are covered by an employer, which amounts to about one-third of all inpatient hospital costs.

This may sound good. But the problem with such plans is that they are viable while you are permanently employed by a specific organization. Freelancers and other part-time workers do not get this coverage. That means that this kind of coverage comes at the cost of personal freedom.

Suppose you are lucky enough to have an employer-sponsored insurance plan. In that case, these plans are among the best, covering almost 85 percent of insurance premiums for employees and 75 percent for employees' dependents.

Though that may sound amazing, nothing comes free in this world. In reality, people have to work for that insurance coverage. In addition, those who receive employer-sponsored health insurance tend to receive lower wages when compared to those without such benefits. So if you really look deep, you are working extra hours to pay for that insurance, yet you have limited control over it. The employer is making many decisions on your behalf.

If you really believe you are in a good position because your employer is bearing a more significant chunk of your insurance costs, think twice.

Some of the leading economists in the US suggest that increasing health insurance costs being paid by employers are one of the most significant reasons why wages have not risen considerably for the last two decades in the US. So remember that however things might look, you are ultimately bearing all those massive health insurance costs.

Not only that, but such employer-sponsored health insurance may also be disrupted if you decide to change jobs, meaning you will face certain troubles when changing careers.

Things are not as rosy if we consider that the number of organizations providing retiree health benefits has been declining consistently since 1980. It has fallen from 66 percent at the peak to below 33 percent.

That is not all. If a small firm employs you, chances are slim that you will get good employee health insurance. Here, the trend is also downward—the number of small firms providing health insurance has been declining since the late 1990s.

Finally, there are individually purchased plans. They used to be the most expensive option. Nonetheless, about 10 percent of Americans opt for them. These plans became more affordable after the introduction of the ACA in 2010, as preexisting medical conditions stopped influencing insurance costs, at least in theory.

Types of Medical Insurance

Health care coverage is different depending on how the insurance plan is funded (i.e., whether publicly or privately). However, there is another way of looking at types of medical insurance: how the insurance company compensates or indemnifies health care expenses.

The traditional way of indemnifying health care costs is either paying a percentage of the provider's fee or paying some fixed amount for each procedure (fee-for-service, or FFS), with the rest of the costs borne by the patient.

FFS plans are traditional health insurance models that typically involve the insurer paying a portion of the health care provider's fee, with the patient covering the remaining cost.

This model offers flexibility in choosing health care providers and services but often involves higher out-of-pocket expenses for the patient. While FFS plans can cover a significant portion of health care costs, they rarely cover everything, making out-of-pocket payments a notable aspect of this model. Despite this, FFS remains popular due to its straightforward approach and wide acceptance among various health care providers.

Another, quite different, kind of model for indemnifying health care expenses is one called a health maintenance organization

(HMO). In this model, all payments for procedures or treatment are directly made to the health care provider, and thus the patient is not involved in the payment process.

However, in the case of HMOs, insurance companies often work with specific clinics and doctors. In addition, they either employ health care providers or have a contract with specific providers. Thus, your insurance will not work everywhere; it will only work in clinics affiliated with the HMO.

Further, this model has a list of conditions covered as their employed or contracted health care providers cannot, in fact, provide all kinds of services. The lack of specific health services or procedures is the limiting factor in these insurance policies. HMOs are part of so-called managed care, a model that helps reduce health care costs. It reduces health care costs by limiting services to a predefined network of providers for a set fee. This model emphasizes cost-efficiency and preventive care but restricts access to certain specialized treatments, defining its primary limitation.

However, there is more to this topic, and you may come across various other terms and approaches for managing health care expenses. Some models blend elements of both traditional fee-for-service health care and managed care, creating hybrid models.

One such example is network-based managed care. In this model, you can benefit from lower treatment costs if you receive care from a designated network of health care providers. Conversely, if you seek treatment outside of this network, you can expect significantly higher fees.

Furthermore, there is a variety of other insurance types beyond these models. For instance, a high-deductible health plan (HDHP) doesn't cover routine medical procedures but is designed to assist with emergencies and high-cost medical treatments exclusively. A limited benefit plan operates differently by providing coverage for minor health issues while capping the annual payout at a specific amount, often not exceeding $2,000.

In addition to the abovementioned insurance categories, there are also nonmedical health insurance policies. These encompass options like disability income insurance and long-term care insurance, which serve different purposes and cater to specific health care needs.

So, yes, understanding the various types of insurance is quite challenging. There are so many that it can be confusing and require much effort and research.

Even worse, health insurance plans often do not cover all your health needs, and you often end up paying out of pocket. As there is no way to predict what health condition may affect you, people often feel cheated by certain insurance companies or feel that the plan did not help them sufficiently.

Yet learning a type of exercise is, relatively speaking, effortless. So if you think that exercising is difficult, think twice. If you develop some health condition, it may be too late. That is why we keep repeating that exercise is the best health insurance. It never cheats you. Even a single step taken is worth it.

END-OF-MODULE-VI ACTIVITIES

Health Insurance Reflection and Planning

Reflection on the Health Care System: Take a moment to reflect on the information presented in this module. Consider the challenges and complexities of the US health care system and its insurance landscape. How do you perceive the current state of health care in the US based on what you've learned?

_____

_____

_____

_____

_____

_____

_____

_____

_____

_____

Personal Health Insurance Assessment: Assess your own health insurance situation. Do you currently have health insurance? If so, is it a public or private plan? Are you satisfied with your coverage, or do you feel there are gaps? Reflect on your insurance experience and any challenges you may have faced.

_____

_____

_____

_____

_____

_____

_____

_____

_____

_____

_____

_____

Improvement and Planning: Based on your reflection, think about potential improvements in the US health care and insurance systems. What changes would you like to see to make health care more accessible and affordable for all?

Your Health and Well-Being: In light of the module's emphasis on the importance of personal health, consider your own well-being. Are you engaging in regular exercise and maintaining a healthy lifestyle? If not, what steps can you take to improve your health and reduce the need for extensive health insurance coverage?

END-OF-MODULE QUIZ

1. **Question:** What percentage of Americans are covered by employer-sponsored insurance?

   A) About 10 percent

   B) Around 33 percent

   C) Approximately 60 percent

   D) Less than 1 percent

2. **Question:** Which public health care program primarily serves individuals aged sixty-five and older?

   A) Medicaid

   B) CHIP

   C) TRICARE

   D) Medicare

3. **Question:** In which model of indemnifying health care expenses is the patient not involved in payment processes, with payments made directly to the health care provider?

   A) Fee-for-service (FFS)

   B) Health Maintenance Organization (HMO)

C) Network-based managed care

D) High-deductible health plan (HDHP)

4. **Question:** What is the primary reason why employer-sponsored health insurance might be considered a double-edged sword?

A) It offers limited coverage.

B) It can lead to lower wages.

C) It doesn't provide any benefits.

D) It is inaccessible to freelancers.

5. **Question:** Why is exercising often emphasized as the best health insurance in the module?

A) Because it is affordable for everyone.

B) Because it doesn't require any effort.

C) Because it can prevent health issues.

D) Because it covers all healthcare expenses.

ANSWERS

1. C) Approximately 60 percent

2. D) Medicare

3. B) Health Maintenance Organization (HMO)

4. B) It can lead to lower wages.

5. C) Because it can prevent health issues.

MODULE VII

HEALTH INSURANCE COMPANIES ARE TRACKING YOUR DATA

If you think your health insurance company is not watching you, you are just too naive. Of course, health insurance companies share patient data with each other and get information from doctors about your health. That is all too obvious.

However, they have other means of tracking you. Many such means are a kind of commercial or trade secret of the companies. Even people working in these insurance firms might not know how these multibillion-dollar corporations track your data. Only a few high-level managers know the reality. These are closely guarded secrets.

Ultimately, the data that insurance companies source from various firms determines the price of your insurance premiums.

Of course, data sharing is quite a complicated science, and it is not done in the way most people imagine.

For example, if you use a specific website to buy supplements, it is never going to share your personal details, such as what you purchased, how often you purchased the items, and other information. Because sharing such details is against the law, these sites need to respect your privacy.

However, people forget that the same website can merely share the data of people whom their AI flagged as individuals quite likely to have a cardiovascular disorder. So, what the organizations do is repack the data in a different format so that they can sell and make money and yet not break any privacy-related laws.

Further, much data leakage is happening even without your consent. Just search for, let's say, omega-3 fatty acids a few times, and you will start seeing online ads related to them. Again, though, everyone is telling you that your personal information is secure with them, and they do not share it with anyone.

More worrisome is the numerous ways your activity is tracked without you even being aware.

Take the example above. You searched the term "omega-3 bene-fits for heart health." So Google searched the term for you and fixed that information within your profile. Is that all? Of course not.

It would be wise to notice that your browser is also tracking your search habits and profiling you. You then get emails that are themselves secure, but some servers are analyzing email headers to understand their content and learn about your routines and health.

When you ultimately ordered the omega-3, you used your debit or credit card. The issuing bank got information about the nature of the transaction, the product supplier also got some in-formation about you, and even UPS or FedEx got a chunk of your health information.

Most people cannot even imagine the number of ways they are being tracked. For example, your phone knows how you move, and your wearables save your health data in the cloud, which can be analyzed.

All this means that IT companies know more about you than you can imagine. Based on this massive amount of information, they prepare your psychological profile and health profile, then use it to market services and products to you or sell that data to larger corporations.

That is why large corporations are providing so many free services to you: for them, your data is the primary source of income.

As we already said, most of these large IT firms do not share the exact data; thus, your detailed information is private. However, they can repack that data in a format that is legal to sell. That is to say, instead of selling precise details on what you bought or searched, they create your profile, which contains your preferences, physical health profile, and more.

Such databases cost massive amounts, and large corporations can afford them as they know that, ultimately, they can make more money by using these tools. For them, your data is just a business tool, and you are an income source.

Hence, a person sitting at the front desk of the insurance company will never see many details about you. But that person will see what category of a client you are. The system may show that you are a high-risk client, and thus you need to pay a higher insurance premium.

Not only that, but the person sitting at the front desk will also not have any power to give you a discount or reduce the price of your health insurance premiums. That is because, based on your profile, some of the options will be blocked on the worker's computer. So even if that person wants to reduce health insurance prices for you, they cannot do it.

What we have said above is just the tip of the iceberg. There is a massive amount of data about us circulating all around.

We are living in the age of the Internet of Things (IoT). Regretfully, this means reduced privacy with each passing day. Smart lamps, smart dishwashers, and smart washing machines sound good. But these gadgets are continually learning about you. They know how active or inactive you were in the last week. They know some things about you better than your close relatives and friends.

After all, chances are slim that your close friends know about your physical activity level, average heart rate, or in which rooms you spend more time in your house. There is no way they can learn much about your spending habits. But unknown individuals know all this information and are tracking you.

So, next time you learn that you need to pay a higher price for your insurance premium, do not be surprised. First, you must understand that data about you are being shared. As we said, they are cleverly repackaged to avoid legal issues.

And let us be realistic. There is not much one can do about all this. You cannot stop using the internet, a smart TV, an Android phone, or debit and credit cards. You cannot stop traveling by car or buying fuel. You also cannot stop buying essential items. So what is the way out? Exercise and exercise.

Our intent is not to frighten you. There are also advantages to this technology. For example, many people feel cheated when they pay massive insurance premiums but have not used any health care services for decades as they are working hard on their health, training, sweating, spending time in the gym, and going through pain.

So look at the positive side of technology too. It can also help save lots of money. If you exercise, buy healthy food products, and have a healthy lifestyle, you will ultimately start paying less for insurance premiums, as the system will show you as a healthy individual or low-risk client.

Thus, instead of wasting time trying to fight a system that was created for a reason, try to understand how it works and use it in your favor.

Remember that if you join exercise boot camp and order healthy foods and supplements, everything is being recorded, and your profile is being continually updated. Thus, exercise can directly impact what you pay for your insurance.

Everything is being tracked: what you eat, where you eat, even the kind of foods you order, how often you go to restaurants, and what kinds of places you prefer to eat. Your exercise preferences, your health conditions, and the medications you use are no exceptions. Nothing is secret.

In most cases, these data are used positively to serve you better and provide you with better options for cost optimization. However, these data may sometimes start working against you, especially if something goes wrong with your health.

END-OF-MODULE-VII ACTIVITIES

Data Awareness and Health Improvement

Reflect on Data Awareness: Take a moment to reflect on the information provided in this module. How does it make you feel knowing that various organizations collect and analyze your data, including your health and lifestyle habits? Are you surprised by the extent of data tracking? Or did you have prior awareness of this?

_____

_____

_____

_____

_____

_____

_____

_____

_____

_____

Data Review: Consider your own online and offline activities. Are there aspects of your life that you are aware could be tracked or analyzed by organizations or technology?

_____

_____

_____

_____

_____

_____

_____

_____

_____

_____

_____

_____

_____

_____

Health and Lifestyle Audit: Conduct a self-audit of your current health and lifestyle habits. Are you satisfied with your exercise routine, dietary choices, and overall well-being? Identify areas where you could make positive changes to improve your health.

Setting Health Goals: Based on your self-audit, set one or two specific health goals. These could be related to increasing your physical activity, improving your diet, or making other lifestyle changes. Ensure these goals are achievable and realistic.

_____

_____

_____

_____

_____

_____

_____

_____

_____

_____

_____

_____

_____

_____

Action Plan: Develop a simple action plan to work toward your health goals. Break down your plan into manageable steps. For example, if your goal is to exercise more, specify the type of exercise, frequency, and duration.

_____

_____

_____

_____

_____

_____

_____

_____

_____

_____

_____

_____

_____

END-OF-MODULE QUIZ

1. **Question:** What is one way health insurance companies use data about individuals?

   A) They share precise details on purchases and searches.

   B) They create psychological profiles.

   C) They provide free services to individuals.

   D) They don't use data for decision-making.

2. **Question:** How do organizations repackage and utilize data legally?

   A) By sharing personal details directly

   B) By breaking privacy-related laws

   C) By creating profiles that mention preferences and health profiles

   D) By selling data without any modifications.

3. **Question:** According to the module, what can individuals do to potentially reduce their insurance premiums?

   A) Stop using technology and the internet

   B) Exercise regularly and maintain a healthy lifestyle

C) File complaints against insurance companies

D) Share more personal data

4. **Question:** How does the module suggest individuals can use technology in their favor regarding insurance premiums?

A) By avoiding all technology use

B) By joining exercise boot camps

C) By not ordering healthy food and supplements

D) By resisting data tracking

5. **Question:** What does the module encourage individuals to do regarding data tracking?

A) Fight against data tracking

B) Understand how data tracking works and use it to their advantage

C) Stop using the internet and technology

D) Share more personal data

ANSWERS

1. B) They create psychological profiles.

2. C) By creating profiles that mention preferences and health profiles

3. B) Exercise regularly and maintain a healthy lifestyle

4. B) By joining exercise boot camps

5. B) Understand how data tracking works and use it to their advantage

MODULE VIII

LIFE AND HEALTH

OK, enough frightening you about data tracking by various firms and privacy issues in the modern world. That may be alarming a bit, but nothing is as bad as being ill. So exercise is not merely about saving on bills. It is more about staying healthy.

Life is a journey from time x to time y, but how enjoyable the journey will be depends on your health. With exercise, you can not only ensure that this journey is pleasant but also prolong the journey.

That is why we call exercise the best health insurance, not life insurance. Life insurance is quite a different thing. It is generally compensation that your loved ones get in the event of your untimely demise. However, you reap the benefits of health insurance during your life.

Still, to reap those benefits, you must be healthy and mentally alert. A bleak soul cannot gain much from life and health.

Without going much into philosophy or spirituality, we all know that humans are not immortal. Hence, it is vital to make the best of whatever time we have in our lives. And everything depends on health, which is a function of how much you move or exercise.

Ultimately, most of the things you achieve in life are directly or indirectly tied to your health and well-being. For example, an unhealthy body cannot produce much wealth, and all the money in the world becomes meaningless for an ailing body.

So start treating your body as something sacred. It is the most precious thing you have. If you take care of your body, additional worldly pleasures will follow. Only health can guarantee different pleasurable moments come to your life, and you can experience them, too.

There has been a lot of research on these topics in the last few decades, and almost every study has concluded that there are just two things that individuals must do to improve their lives: *exercise and take dietary measures.*

Genetics cannot change much during your lifetime, though it may change a bit, and even that is possible through exercise. The environment in which we live can be enhanced, but we all must work together.

That said, each individual has the power to make substantial improvements in their life expectancy and overall health by paying attention to their dietary choices and physical activity.

When considering the two most critical factors for human life and health, diet and exercise come to mind. First, it's evident that one cannot survive without food—that's a well-established fact. But the distinction lies in consuming a healthy, balanced diet.

After food, if there is anything else one can do to promote health and well-being, it is exercise. Yet, regretfully, it is among the neglected elements of life. Most people are still not exercising regularly.

When someone has not eaten for a long time, they become hungry, and their body demands food. In other words, the body will let you know.

However, signals of the need for exercise are more subtle. Though they are there, many people fail to react to them. This is, perhaps, unlike food deficit, which may affect your health quickly.

Lack of exercise, on the other hand, causes health damage over a prolonged period.

Of course, there are other reasons why many people neglect exercise. For example, consuming food is more pleasurable than strenuous physical activity. Although, once you get used to exercise, it may also become enjoyable and a habit, but that requires time and dedication.

It is also worth noticing that food sometimes harms you. This is because finding sufficient food has been a challenge for thousands of years. Hence, humans have evolved to consume a great deal of food if it is available in abundance.

On the other hand, many people associate physical activity with some discomfort. As a result, they become sedentary, and they lose the ability to carry out physical movements properly, and then they realize that they have lost some precious ability.

Again, to stay healthy, have a well-balanced diet and exercise regularly. Of course, one can experience more significant health benefits by combining exercise with specific dietary measures. These two measures are not mutually exclusive but rather complement each other.

Exercise and dietary measures together can ensure good health for a long time. If you pay attention to these two factors, it is pretty likely that you will rarely fall ill.

Lower Your Insurance and Medical Expenses with Diet and Exercise

Till now, we have mainly focused on how regular exercise can benefit health in numerous ways. However, when you add exercise to dietary measures, you will experience much more significant gains and positive health effects.

Eating a balanced diet, sleep, and exercise are three simple and effective ways to achieve good health. Among them, eating a balanced diet and exercise require relatively more significant planning and understanding. However, if the balance between these three activities is maintained, it will translate into reduced insurance payments, reduced medical expenses, and good health.

Though sleep is self-explanatory, diet and exercise are not. Of course, unlike in the case of exercise, there is no chance that someone will forget to eat. However, the problem these days is not sufficient consumption of food or calories but rather dietary imbalances.

A sedentary lifestyle not only makes you physically weak but also influences your dietary choices. For example, those who do not exercise are less likely to think about what they eat. Even worse, they are more likely to consume high-calorie foods and foods with a poor nutritional profile.

Surely, fries can provide massive amounts of calories. However, they mainly contain poor-quality fats and fast-absorbing carbs. In addition, they have almost no protein content and very few vitamins.

So, if you aspire to lead a healthy life, it's essential to understand that a significant part of it hinges on maintaining a balanced diet and engaging in regular exercise. While this book primarily focuses on exercise, it's crucial to acknowledge that diet and exercise are interconnected. A poorly structured diet can offset the potential health benefits of exercise.

Many foods that we consume on a daily basis are delicious and addictive, contain massive amounts of calories, and yet have very few vital nutrients. Burning those extra calories requires much effort. For example, a one-hour moderate-intensity workout is barely enough to burn the calories in a bar of chocolate.

We're certainly not implying that you should completely eliminate specific foods from your diet. Rather, it's important to recognize that certain foods are best consumed in moderation.

Dietary planning does not require massive amounts of time and effort. It only requires some understanding of the basics of what the human body needs to stay healthy.

If you want to stay healthy and enjoy the greatest benefits of good health, you do not need to switch to some specific diet. Just a few simple measures can help significantly. For example, avoid ultraprocessed foods or foods that are the product of industrialization. Instead, buy fresh foods and cook for yourself. That is one of the simplest ways to shed body weight and improve quality of life. Unfortunately, most calorie-dense foods are ultraprocessed foods.

The problem is not so much in the foods but in how they are made. Some data suggest that people in Western countries are getting almost 70 percent of their calories from ultraprocessed foods. These are comfort foods, and most of these foods are ready to eat or require minimum preparatory work.

But if you want to save on health insurance, start cooking more frequently. Instead of canned foods or sausages, think about chicken soup, apples, and berries. You do not have to sacrifice much. All you need to do is change your food choices.

Most dietary measures work because they force people to make significant changes in the way they eat. Just think of paleo, DASH, keto, Atkin's, and other diet forms. They force you to avoid some foods and start thinking about what goes into your body. These diets are not essentially about fasting. They are, rather, about changing your food habits.

You can become healthy even without practicing any specific diet form. For example, the DASH diet is not a diet form in the real sense. It is just a bunch of instructions regarding what to avoid and what to eat more frequently.

As mentioned earlier, our intention is not to prescribe a specific dietary plan but to promote awareness. While exercise is indeed pivotal for good health, dietary choices can complement and enhance its effects.

The truth is that those who eat mindfully and exercise rarely develop chronic health issues. Such individuals might sometimes contract a seasonal infection or have an accident. Even then, they make a quick comeback and don't need to pay massive medical bills. Thus, they do not need to worry too much about their insurance.

With the right kind of dietary approach and exercise program, you might not only slow down aging but also reduce your metabolic age. That is the reason why you are much less likely to fall ill.

Theoretically, exercise can help you travel back in time! In most cases, it is possible to reduce your metabolic age by as many as ten years. Generally, reducing metabolic age by three to five years with moderate exercise is not challenging. However, to achieve more significant results, you must also take dietary measures.

Finally, remember that when we talk about exercise, we are not just referring to physical activity. Over the long run, your aim must be to switch to a healthier lifestyle. That means giving up smoking, reducing your caffeine intake, minimizing alcohol intake, keeping your body hydrated, and ensuring adequate intake of micronutrients.

What you need to do is adopt a healthy lifestyle. However, starting to exercise might be the primary way to start making global changes in lifestyle.

For example, if you think that you will start exercising after quitting smoking or giving up alcohol completely, it may not work. Harmful habits are not an excuse to delay getting started with exercise.

Instead, remember that once you start exercising, you will realize that many things become much easier for you, including giving up substance abuse and other harmful habits.

As we have already mentioned, exercise causes changes in your brain and improves your mental health. Thus, exercise increases your willpower and ability to make decisions. It also reduces addiction, and when you exercise, you stop enjoying harmful foods, alcohol, smoking, caffeine, and more.

Exercise is among the biggest self-confidence and self-esteem enhancers. Moreover, if you stick to it for long enough, it will result in a complete transformation.

Remember that there will be periods of discouragement when you will feel as if you are not making any progress. However, one pretty day, you will realize that somehow, suddenly, much has changed inside you. Basically, progress does not occur linearly; instead, you are more likely to make a quantum jump.

Take this example: When you try to memorize something, you may find it hard and fail to remember the information even after repeating it several times. But then, you take a break and come back only to realize that it now takes much less effort to memorize the information or solve the problem. That is because progress is more likely to occur in quantum jumps.

Similarly, when you exercise, there will be periods when you will not notice much health improvement. If you stick to your exercise program and tweak it if needed, however, one day, you will suddenly realize that something has changed amazingly and in quite a short time.

To sum up, there are millions of health benefits of exercise. In addition, it can significantly reduce your medical bills and insurance premium.

Although there are many types of insurance plans, and their cost depends on numerous factors, for an average person living in the US, health insurance cost equates to 10-20 percent of annual income. Yes, that is a massive amount.

If you do some math, you find that means each year, a person has to work for a month and a half or even two months just to cover insurance costs! Or, if you work forty hours a week, you work half a day or even one full day a week just to pay for your health insurance.

Of course, you won't be able to nullify your insurance costs (which we don't recommend in the first place), but you can at least reduce the number of hours you work for insurance each week. However, whether you need to work four hours a week or eight to cover your insurance costs depends on your health status.

Wouldn't it be better to work about four hours a week (10 percent of the workweek) to cover your insurance costs and spend the other four hours exercising? After all, working extra hours for medical bills or insurance will not make you a healthy or happy person. On the other hand, spending three to six hours working out each week can make a massive difference. It helps save on medical bills and insurance and makes you a much happier and healthier person.

If you do the calculations, it is not difficult to see that exercise is quite a beneficial activity. Moreover, once you start exercising, it starts justifying itself, resulting in increased returns in every way, whether financial, psychological, or spiritual.

That is why we say that exercise is the best insurance.

END-OF-MODULE-VIII ACTIVITIES

Exercise and Diet Journaling Challenge

Personal Reflection: Take a moment to reflect on your current exercise habits and dietary choices. Are you exercising regularly, occasionally, or not at all? How would you rate your current diet in terms of its nutritional quality?

_____

_____

_____

_____

_____

_____

_____

_____

_____

_____

_____

Exercise and Diet Planner: Based on your reflection, set some fitness goals and dietary intentions for the next month. Be specific about the number of days you plan to exercise each week and any dietary changes you want to make.

_____

_____

_____

_____

_____

_____

_____

_____

_____

_____

_____

_____

_____

Implementation: Put your exercise and diet plan into action for a month. Stick to your exercise schedule and make an effort to follow your dietary intentions. Pay attention to how you feel physically and mentally during this period.

Daily Journaling: Keep a daily journal to record your exercise activities, including the type of exercise, duration, and any notes about how you felt during and after the session. Additionally, document your daily dietary choices, mentioning what you ate and any observations about your eating habits.

Reflection and Adjustment: At the end of the month, review your exercise and diet journal. Reflect on your achievements, any challenges you faced, and how your health and well-being have been affected. Adjust your exercise and diet plan for the next month based on your reflections.

END-OF-MODULE QUIZ

1. **Question:** What are the two fundamental factors that individuals can focus on to improve their health and well-being?

   A) Sleep and social interaction

   B) Exercise and dietary choices

   C) Meditation and medication

   D) Television and technology

2. **Question:** Why is dietary planning important in conjunction with exercise?

   A) It helps you lose weight faster,

   B) It complements and enhances the benefits of exercise,

   C) It makes exercise unnecessary.

   D) It has no impact on health.

3. **Question:** Which of the following statements regarding dietary choices and exercise is true?

   A) Exercise can compensate for an unhealthy diet.

   B) Dietary choices have no effect on health.

C) A well-balanced diet can offset the benefits of exercise.

D) Diet and exercise work together to promote good health.

4. **Question:** What is one common challenge people face in maintaining a healthy diet when they don't exercise regularly?

A) They become better at cooking.

B) They develop a strong craving for unhealthy foods.

C) They start enjoying strenuous physical activity.

D) They pay more attention to their dietary choices.

5. **Question:** Which of the following is not a benefit of regular exercise?

A) Improved physical health

B) Increased willpower and decision-making abilities

C) Enhanced self-confidence and self-esteem

D) Reduction in the need for sleep

ANSWERS:

1. B) Exercise and dietary choices
2. B) It complements and enhances the benefits of exercise
3. D) Diet and exercise work together to promote good health
4. B) T   hey develop a strong craving for unhealthy foods
5. D) Reduction in the need for sleep

REFERENCES

[1] "Leading Causes of Death," September 6, 2022. https://www.cdc.gov/nchs/fastats/leading-causes-of-death.html (accessed December 1, 2022).

[2] B. W. Wu et al., "Genotype vs. Phenotype and the Rise of Non-Communicable Diseases: The Importance of Lifestyle Behaviors During Childhood," *Cureus*, vol. 8, no. 1, p. e458, doi: 10.7759/cureus.458.

[3] "Symptoms & Causes of Diabetes | NIDDK," *National Institute of Diabetes and Digestive and Kidney Diseases.* https://www.niddk.nih.gov/health-information/diabetes/overview/symptoms-causes (accessed December 1, 2022).

[4] "Facts About Chronic Kidney Disease," *National Kidney Foundation*, May 15, 2020. https://www.kidney.org/atoz/content/about-chronic-kidney-disease (accessed December 1, 2022).

[5] G. S. Wander and M. Bansal, "Legacy effect in medicine—the expanding horizon" *Indian Heart J*, vol. 70, no. 6, pp. 769–771, 2018, doi: 10.1016/j.ihj.2018.12.001.

[6] "Dementia." https://www.who.int/news-room/fact-sheets/detail/dementia (accessed December 1, 2022).

[7] E. W. Gregg and A. Menke, "Diabetes and Disability," in *Diabetes in America*, 3rd ed., C. C. Cowie, S. S. Casagrande, A. Menke, M. A. Cissell, M. S. Eberhardt, J. B. Meigs, E. W. Gregg, W. C. Knowler, E. Barrett-Connor, D. J. Becker, F. L. Brancati, E. J. Boyko, W. H. Herman, B. V. Howard, K. M. V. Narayan, M. Rewers, and J. E. Fradkin, eds. Bethesda (MD): National Institute of Diabetes and Digestive and Kidney Diseases, 2018. http://www.ncbi.nlm.nih.gov/books/NBK567983/ (accessed December 1, 2022).

[8] A. Sharma, V. Madaan, and F. D. Petty, "Exercise for Mental Health," *Prim Care Companion J Clin Psychiatry*, vol. 8, no. 2, p. 106, 2006.

[9] E. Hacker, "Exercise and Quality of Life: Strengthening the Connections," *Clin J Oncol Nurs*, vol. 13, no. 1, pp. 31–39, February 2009, doi: 10.1188/09.CJON.31-39.

[10] D. J. Mersy, "Health benefits of aerobic exercise," *Postgrad Med*, vol. 90, no. 1, pp. 103–107, 110–112, July 1991, doi: 10.1080/00325481.1991.11700983.

[11] "American Heart Association Recommendations for Physical Activity in Adults and Kids," www.heart.org. https://*www. heart.org*/en/healthy-living/fitness/fitness-basics/aha-recs-for-physical-activity-in-adults (accessed December 1, 2022).

[12] "Target Heart Rate and Estimated Maximum Heart Rate | Physical Activity | CDC," October 20, 2022. https://www.cdc.gov/physicalactivity/basics/measuring/heartrate.htm (accessed December 1, 2022).

[13] Department of Health and Human Services, "Resistance training—health benefits." http://www.betterhealth.vic.gov.au/health/healthyliving/resistance-training-health-benefits (accessed December 1, 2022).

[14] K. R. Hirsch et al., "Metabolic effects of high-intensity interval training and essential amino acids," *Eur J Appl Physiol*, vol.
121, no. 12, pp. 3297–3311, December 2021, doi: 10.1007/
s00421-021-04792-4.

[15] F. Li, P. Harmer, E. Eckstrom, K. Fitzgerald, L.-S. Chou,
and Y. Liu, "Effectiveness of Tai Ji Quan vs Multimodal and
Stretching Exercise Interventions for Reducing Injurious Falls
in Older Adults at High Risk of Falling: Follow-up Analysis
of a Randomized Clinical Trial," *JAMA Network Open*,
vol. 2, no. 2, p. e188280, February 2019, doi: 10.1001/
jamanetworkopen.2018.8280.

[16] M. D. Klok, S. Jakobsdottir, and M. L. Drent, "The role of
leptin and ghrelin in the regulation of food intake and body
weight in humans: a review," *Obes Rev*, vol. 8, no. 1, pp. 21–
34, January 2007, doi: 10.1111/j.1467-789X.2006.00270.x.

[17] N. A. King, A. Tremblay, and J. E. Blundell, "Effects of exercise on appetite control: implications for energy balance,"
Med Sci Sports Exerc, vol. 29, no. 8, pp. 1076–1089, August
1997, doi: 10.1097/00005768-199708000-00014.

[18] S. Christie, G. A. Wittert, H. Li, and A. J. Page, "Involvement of TRPV1 Channels in Energy Homeostasis," *Front Endocrinol (Lausanne)*, vol. 9, p. 420, July 2018, doi: 10.3389/fendo. 2018.00420.

[19] S. F. McCarthy, H. Islam, and T. J. Hazell, "The emerging role of lactate as a mediator of exercise-induced appetite suppression," *American Journal of Physiology-Endocrinology and Metabolism*, vol. 319, no. 4, pp. E814–E819, October 2020, doi: 10.1152/ajpendo.00256.2020.

[20] CDC, "Obesity is a Common, Serious, and Costly Disease," *Centers for Disease Control and Prevention*, July 20, 2022. https://www.cdc.gov/obesity/data/adult.html (accessed December 01, 2022).

[21] H. Rosen, "Is Obesity A Disease or A Behavior Abnormality? Did the AMA Get It Right?" *Mo Med*, vol. 111, no. 2, pp. 104–108, 2014.

[22] "National Diabetes Statistics Report | Diabetes | CDC," June 29, 2022. https://www.cdc.gov/diabetes/data/statistics-report/index.html (accessed December 1, 2022).

[23] R. R. Wing et al., "Benefits of Modest Weight Loss in Improving Cardiovascular Risk Factors in Overweight and Obese Individuals With Type 2 Diabetes," *Diabetes Care*, vol. 34, no. 7, pp. 1481–1486, July 2011, doi: 10.2337/dc10-2415.

[24] J. P. H. Wilding, "The importance of weight management in type 2 diabetes mellitus," *Int J Clin Pract*, vol. 68, no. 6, pp. 682–691, June 2014, doi: 10.1111/ijcp.12384.

[25] C. Hearing, W. Chang, K. Szuhany, T. Deckersbach, A. Nierenberg, and L. Sylvia, "Physical Exercise for Treatment of Mood Disorders: A Critical Review," *Curr Behav Neurosci Rep*, vol. 3, no. 4, pp. 350–359, December 2016, doi: 10.1007/s40473-016-0089-y.

[26] S. Nazarpour, M. Simbar, F. Ramezani Tehrani, and H. Alavi Majd, "Sexual Function and Exercise in Postmenopausal Women Residing in Chalous and Nowshahr, Northern Iran," *Iran Red Crescent Med J*, vol. 18, no. 5, p. e30120, January 2016, doi: 10.5812/ircmj.30120.

[27] "Four Types of Exercise Can Improve Your Health and Physical Ability," *National Institute on Aging.* https://www.nia.nih.gov/health/four-types-exercise-can-improve-your-health-and-physical-ability (accessed December 1, 2022).

[28] H. Ihira et al., "Association Between Physical Activity and Risk of Disabling Dementia in Japan," *JAMA Network Open*, vol. 5, no. 3, p. e224590, March 2022, doi: 10.1001/jamanetworkopen.2022.4590.

[29] "Benefits of Exercise for Osteoarthritis | Arthritis Foundation." https://www.arthritis.org/health-wellness/healthy-living/physical-activity/getting-started/benefits-of-exercise-for-osteoarthritis (accessed December 1, 2022).

ACKNOWLEDGMENTS

As I sit down to pen these acknowledgments, my heart is filled with profound gratitude for each individual who contributed to the fruition of this book. This journey, much like the essence of the book—the transformative power of exercise and a healthy lifestyle—has been a profound learning experience.

First and foremost, my deepest thanks are extended to the myriad health care professionals, fitness experts, and nutritionists who contributed to this work. Their willingness to share their profound knowledge and insights has been the cornerstone of the book, making it not just a source of information but a practical guide for a healthier life.

The invaluable input and meticulous scrutiny provided by the peer reviewers have been pivotal. Their critical evaluations and insightful feedback have greatly elevated the quality and precision of the content.

To my family and friends, your unwavering support and endless patience have been my pillars of strength. The countless hours spent writing and revising this book would have been insurmountable without your constant encouragement and understanding.

A special thanks to the editorial team and our publishers. Your expertise, guidance, and unrelenting commitment have been vital in transforming a vision into reality. Further, your dedication to maintaining high standards of professionalism has been crucial in making this book accessible and engaging.

And to you, the readers, my deepest gratitude. Your quest for better health and well-being is not only commendable but also the very inspiration behind this book. It is my earnest hope that the insights shared here will be a valuable guide in your journey toward a more vibrant and fulfilling life.

In conclusion, this book is a testament to the power of collaboration in spreading knowledge and empowerment. I hope it acts as a beacon of positive change in your lives and keeps the flame of learning and personal growth alive.

With heartfelt thanks,
Wisler Saint-Vil, MD, MBA